Competency in Healthcare

a practical guide to competency frameworks

Les Storey

John Howard

and

Alan Gillies

Radcliffe Medical Press

Radcliffe Medical Press Ltd
18 Marcham Road
Abingdon
Oxon OX14 1AA
United Kingdom

www.radcliffe-oxford.com
The Radcliffe Medical Press electronic catalogue and online ordering facility.
Direct sales to anywhere in the world.

British Library Cataloguing in Publication Data

A catalogue record for this book is available from the British Library.

ISBN 1 85775 926 5

Typeset by Joshua Associates Ltd, Oxford
Printed and bound by TJ International Ltd, Padstow, Cornwall

Contents

Why you should read this book

The purpose of this book is to help you ensure that your staff have the skills they need to carry out their job properly. It is also about being able to demonstrate this. In the current environment dominated by scandal and the clinical governance agenda, the latter may be at least as important as the former.

By the time you have read this book, you should understand:

- what a competency framework is
- how such a framework can be defined
- how such a framework can be implemented
- how such a framework can be used to help an organisation
- how such a framework can be combined with models of organisational development
- how such models can be computerised.

We hope that you enjoy reading it as well!

Les Storey
lstorey@uclan.ac.uk

John Howard
jhoward1@uclan.ac.uk

Alan Gillies
acgillies@uclan.ac.uk

July 2002

About the authors

Les Storey
Senior Lecturer
Faculty of Health
University of Central Lancashire

John Howard
Senior Lecturer in Health Informatics
Health Informatics Research Unit
Lancashire Postgraduate School of Medicine and Health
University of Central Lancashire

Alan Gillies
Professor of Information Management
Health Informatics Research Unit
University of Central Lancashire

Acknowledgements

The authors would like to acknowledge the help and support provided by individuals and organisations in developing the model and frameworks described in this book.

These include:

- Ashworth Hospital Authority
- Blackburn, Hyndburn and Ribble Valley NHS Trust
- Colin Dale.

1

Competence and competency

Introduction

Throughout healthcare the competences required to provide an effective service to our patients are continually being utilised. When a patient attends a hospital for an out-patient appointment they will encounter many different staff groups, all of whom need a range of competences to do their job. These may include porters, receptionists, care assistants, nurses, doctors, radiographers, physiotherapists, occupational therapists, phlebotomists and pharmacists, to name but a few.

Many of the competences will be common across the disciplines, but the levels of proficiency required to carry out the task may vary. For example, the simple task of communicating with a patient will vary significantly; the porter may be required to give directions to the clinic whilst the nurse, doctor or other healthcare professional may be required to provide complex information to patients who may be distressed and anxious.

Another example would be an individual who is involved in a road traffic accident and as a consequence suffers a broken limb. At all stages of the process of dealing with this patient, different levels of proficiency are needed because of the different contexts within which care is delivered. These include:

- at the scene of the accident
- in the accident and emergency department
- in the radiography department
- in the operating theatre
- on the ward

- in physiotherapy
- at home.

One of the competences that will be common across all of these areas is 'Assess patient's healthcare needs'. At each stage in the care continuum the healthcare professionals involved will need to have the appropriate level of proficiency to deal effectively with the patient and assess their needs:

- the ambulance paramedic
- the receptionist
- the A&E triage nurse
- the senior house officer
- the radiographer
- the operating department assistant
- the theatre nurse
- the surgical registrar
- the anaesthetist
- the recovery-room nurse
- the ward clerk
- the ward nurse
- the consultant
- the healthcare assistant
- the physiotherapist
- the community nurse
- the general practitioner.

In assessing the health needs of the patient at each stage of his care trajectory, different skills, knowledge, understanding and decision-making are required because of the different contexts within which the assessments are taking place. The paramedic will be making assessments of need in conditions that could be dangerous to them and to the patient; they are the first on the scene, delivering emergency aid, prioritising actions and determining the immediate future care needs. In the accident and emergency department the triage nurse will assess needs at another stage; she will identify options available within the department and will plan the throughcare of the patient in A&E.

Whilst in A&E the senior house officer (SHO) will use skills and experience to determine the best means to meet the patient's needs. They will have to decide if they can deal with the patient themselves or if they need to involve more senior medical staff.

Having decided on a course of action, the patient moves on through the radiography department then on to the operating theatre, where choices of treatment are again made; the orthopaedic registrar makes a choice between reduction of the fracture and the use of plaster casts or surgical intervention and pinning and plating the fracture.

And so the process of 'Assess patient's healthcare needs' goes on. It can be seen from these examples that a range of competences are needed to deal with each patient interaction, and that for each of the competences a range of proficiency levels are required by each of the disciplines involved in care delivery.

This book has been compiled as an aid for healthcare practitioners and managers in order to raise awareness of the issue of competence and to provide guidance on how to implement competence frameworks and utilise them as part of a strategic approach to developing a workforce that meets society's healthcare needs.

The book provides a background to competency-based approaches to healthcare, sets the current policy and strategies in context, and gives illustrations of a number of case studies where competency frameworks are being introduced.

The concept of competence

The need for defined competences for healthcare professionals has been clearly articulated by many organisations and authors (Benner 1984; Storey *et al.* 1995a,b; UKCC 1999a,b), including the recently published inquiries at Bristol Royal Infirmary (NHS Executive 2001) and Oxford Cardiac Services (NHS Executive 2000). The emerging competence frameworks and portfolio systems are providing a foundation to support lifelong learning and continuing professional development.

Competency frameworks can also be utilised by employers to develop competency-based job descriptions. Competency-based job descriptions enable employers – and employees – to have a clear understanding of expectations in relation to role performance; they can be used to undertake training needs analysis, contribute to individual performance review, and provide a basis for developing continuing education packages that meet the needs of the service and individual employees.

Despite the significant interest and investment in competence and competency-based education, there are still some barriers to the universal acceptance of outcomes-based approaches to professional nursing education. Competency-based approaches are still seen by some to be less attractive than traditional qualifications and to a certain extent professional and academic snobbery still exists. Another criticism that has been levelled at competency-based approaches is that the assessment processes are sometimes paper-driven and bureaucratic.

However, from the level of activity being undertaken by statutory bodies, including the General Medical Council and UKCC, professional organisations such as the Royal College of General Practitioners and the Royal College of Nursing, education providers and employing organisations, the momentum to develop and implement competency-based approaches to professional development programmes continues to grow. Competency-based approaches provide a mechanism for all key stakeholders in healthcare provision to ensure the quality of the care provided and to contribute to public protection.

Competence can be defined as the ability of the practitioner to practice safely and effectively to a professional standard. And as such the practitioner should be able to determine their level of competence in carrying out particular functions and take measures to develop and maintain competence. To be competent it is not enough to be able to fulfil a particular function; the competent practitioner must have the ability to problem solve, think critically and utilise effective evidence on which to base their practice and work within a multi-disciplinary team.

Competence, higher education and employment

It is generally accepted that until the latter part of the twentieth century the main aim of higher education was to create knowledgeable individuals who by their knowledge had more likelihood of becoming competent. It could be argued whether they actually became competent was outwith the interests of higher education. Educational programmes within higher education are designed to produce graduates who have the capability to become competent practitioners. They instil knowledge, skills and understanding in the students, but will fail to meet the needs of employment if another dimension is missing. That dimension is application. If students cannot apply their knowledge, skills and understanding in the workplace, then education is failing to meet market need (Storey 1998). As we moved towards the twenty-first century the needs of employment became a key issue. This was acknowledged within the United Kingdom when a commission into higher education was established in 1996. Gillian Shepherd, then Secretary of State for Education and Employment, said:

> Today's graduates face a different world from their predecessors. They must be prepared for changes in the nature of work and the

greater demands it makes. Increasingly, they will need to switch career more than once in their lifetime. We must ensure that they are equipped with the skills and flexibility needed by the labour market of the twenty-first century – through both initial education and updating and up-skilling throughout their lives. Higher education must be in the best shape possible to meet these needs . . . As the pace of change quickens, there will be a greater premium on the capacity to innovate . . . Higher education can help too to drive local and regional regeneration through services to employers.

(Shepherd 1996)

Healthcare within the United Kingdom has responded to this challenge with a number of policy documents from the Government and statutory bodies focusing on competency approaches and the need to produce practitioners 'who are fit for practice, fit for purpose and fit for award' (UKCC 1999a). These initiatives have resulted in the development of a new curriculum for pre-registration nursing that is designed:

. . . to prepare the student to provide the nursing care that patients require, safely and competently, and to assume the responsibilities and accountabilities necessary for public protection.

(UKCC 1999a)

The issue of competence in healthcare appears to be a key agenda item in a number of countries, including the Republic of Ireland, the United Kingdom and Australia. The International Council of Nurses (ICN) has acknowledged that because of the developing global market 'there is considerable and legitimate interest, across many regions of the world, in seeking international recognition of the professional qualifications and related competencies of the many different groups of professionals' (ICN 2001). This approach is also relevant to other healthcare professionals. In the allied healthcare professions competency-based approaches have also been introduced, and frameworks of competence have been introduced to support continuing professional development.

In the UK, policy documents from the Department of Health and NHS Executive all make reference to competence and are impacting on the future direction of education and training for healthcare professionals. *The NHS Plan* (DoH 2000a), *A Health Service of all the talents* (DoH 2000b) *Fitness for Practice* (UKCC 1999a), *Standards for a Higher Level of Practice* (UKCC 1999b), *Agenda for Change* (NHS Executive 1999) and *Making a Difference* (DoH 1999) all promote the development of the competence of the healthcare workforce and promote the implementation of a competency/outcomes-based approach to education and practice. In Australia, a commission into nurse education is currently being conducted, and again, one of the key issues relates to the competence of nurses to practice on completion of their pre-registration education programme.

Competency-based approaches to professional education are becoming more common and appear to offer the opportunity to develop flexible programmes that meet needs of students, practitioners and their employers. A recent report commissioned by the UKCC, *Nursing in Secure Environments* (UKCC and University of Central Lancashire 1999), concluded that a competence framework lends itself to the development of modular, competency-based programmes that can be delivered through a number of media. It went on to suggest that classroom-based programmes do not need to be the main method of delivery, and that open and distance-learning packages are available to support such a programme or can be developed. This approach appears to concur with the recommendations in the inquiry into Bristol Royal Infirmary (NHS Executive 2001).

Definitions and types of competence models

A cursory review of the literature reveals that there is no common approach or agreed definition of competence. Without clear direction, there is potential for a number of competence frameworks emerging that may lead to confusion and replication of effort by nurses attempting to meet the requirements of each system.

There is a significant number of definitions and types of competence described in the professional literature, including Hogston (1993) and the Nursing Board for Scotland (1995).

In 1988 the World Health Organization described competence as:

> Competence requires knowledge, appropriate attitudes and observable mechanical or intellectual skills which together account for the ability to deliver a specified professional service.
>
> (WHO 1988, p. 68)

The International Council of Nurses' (1997) definition of competence is:

> A level of performance demonstrating the effective application of knowledge, skill and judgement.

While the Professional and Practice Development Forum Scotland (1997) suggested that:

> Competence, in the context of each practitioner's application of professional judgement and accountability for safe and effective clinical practice, is the ability to continuously demonstrate knowledge and skills against measurable outcomes.

More recently, in 1999 the UKCC Commission for Education created the following definition:

> Competence is the skills and ability to practice safely and effectively without the need for direct supervision.

In 1984, Benner suggested that a competent practitioner is one who sees actions in terms of long-range goals or plans of which she is consciously aware. However, in Benner's view, competence is only one level, and proficiency and expertise go beyond competence.

In the literature, competence is defined in a number of ways. Eraut (2001) defines two types of competence: 'socially defined competence' and 'individually situated competence'. He suggests that:

> *Socially defined competence* is the ability to perform the tasks required to the expected standard.

- Applies to any career stage.
- Expected standard will vary with experience and responsibility.
- Takes into account lifelong learning and changes in 'good practice'.
- Does not specify whose requirements and expectations are to be taken into account.

Individually situated competence is an underlying characteristic of an individual that is causally related to criterion-referenced effective and/or superior performance in a job or situation which:

- is psychometrically derived
- is used for selection or assessment of training needs
- accounts for some variation in performance.

(Eraut 2001)

From the diverse definitions and models of competence it could be argued that competence is still a confusing concept. Competence is seen as an 'absolute' in some definitions whilst it is 'relative' in others. However, there are a number of common themes that are reflected in the definitions of competence. These are:

- knowledge, understanding and judgement
- a range of skills – cognitive, technical or psychomotor, and interpersonal
- a range of personal attributes.

(ICN 2001)

In order to attempt to clarify this confusion it might be worth considering competence as a dynamic process that changes as experience, knowledge and skills develop through and in practice. If we think of a continuum ranging from just knowing how to do something at the one end, to knowing how to do something very well at the other, knowing how to do something competently could fall somewhere along the continuum, and through development of experience and knowledge, competence fluctuates throughout practice.

Mitchell (1998) suggests that competence models can come in a number of forms but can be generalised under the three following types:

- 'what people should be like' – models based on personal characteristics or an individual's behaviour
- 'what people need to possess' – models based on acquiring knowledge, understanding and skills
- 'what people need to achieve in the workplace' – models based on outcomes and standards, including underpinning knowledge and skills.

(Mitchell 1998)

It is the latter model, 'what people need to achieve in the workplace', which appears to be accepted as the preferred model in most organisations and a number of competency frameworks are emerging based on this.

Whichever model of competence is used within professional education programmes, the assessment of competence should include the assessment of cognitive, affective and psychomotor skills. Therefore an aggregated definition of competence could be:

Competence is the knowledge, skills, abilities and behaviours that a practitioner needs to perform their work to a professional standard, and is a key lever for achieving results that will enable the organisation to achieve its healthcare objectives.

Benefits of competence models

The competences needed to undertake a given role in healthcare should prepare practitioners who are fit for purpose and fit to practice. Competences are needed to provide recognition of learning, wherever it takes place, and provide links between individual and organisational requirements, which should enable cost-effective education and training programmes to be delivered.

The issue of competence pervades all professional areas. Much work has been undertaken in the last few years to develop competences or national occupational standards for professionals. These include accountants, engineers, psychologists, social workers, probation officers, health promotion advisors, information management and professions allied to medicine.

In England, NHS Executive-funded projects have been commissioned to develop competence frameworks and examine the relevance of national occupational standards to a range of healthcare professionals, including medicine, radiography and allied health professionals. In addition, the NHS Information Authority has developed a framework of competences that permeate all areas of healthcare.

In nursing, a number of reports have been produced, including *Utilising National Occupational Standards as a Complement to Nursing Curricula* (Storey *et al.* 1995b), *Occupational Standards – A Framework for Clinical Effectiveness?* (O'Hanlon and Andrews 1997) and *Nursing in Secure Environments* (UKCC and University of Central Lancashire 1999). All three reports have concluded that occupational standards 'have much to offer the professions' (O'Hanlon and Andrews 1997), and suggest that national occupational standards 'provide a common language that can be used to describe nursing and articulate clearly expected performance. They also provide a potential national curriculum template that would assist education providers in devising curricula, thus ensuring that nurses completing programmes are "fit for purpose"' (O'Hanlon and Andrews 1997).

National occupational standards are defined by the occupational sector and specify the outcome of work activities. They describe what should happen and what should be achieved and are structured to include:

- **performance criteria:** how you know that the outcome is the right quality
- **range:** situations and contexts to which the standard applies
- **knowledge specification:** what the individual needs to know, understand and apply to achieve the outcome
- **evidence requirements:** types and sources of evidence required to prove that the outcome has has been achieved.

Occupational standards describe in 'ideal' terms what people need to be able to do in employment.

Benefits of competency frameworks

The benefits of developing and implementing competency frameworks have been highlighted by a number of authors, including Eraut (1994 and 1998), Storey *et al.* (1995a, b) and McAllister (1998). Competency frameworks are said to:

- provide a clear picture of the role and responsibilities of the professional
- inform the process of ensuring protection of the public
- facilitate free movement of professionals globally and across national borders
- promote individual and collective professional accountability
- clarify the contribution of the professional *vis-à-vis* the contribution of healthcare and other professionals within the multi-disciplinary team
- provide a foundation for the design of curricula and processes of assessment in both theory and practice settings, which will ensure not only that healthcare professionals are educated and trained to meet current needs for healthcare in their country, but that they are committed to maintaining their competence
- assist in specifying professional expectations associated with roles
- provide a foundation for setting job-specific performance criteria (adapted from ICN 2001).

Delivering competence

The key to 'fitness for purpose' and 'fitness for practice' lies in the ability of education commissioners and purchasers reaching agreement with the education and training providers on the competence outcomes that a student should have acquired, and be able to use in practice, at the end of a programme of learning (Storey *et al.* 1995a, b).

In order to achieve competence in the workplace, professionals must demonstrate this through practice by integrating cognitive, affective and psychomotor skills. It is not inconceivable, therefore, that national occupational standards and/or National Vocational Qualification (NVQ) units might be used as programme outcomes, as in the UK these are part of a nationally accepted framework of qualifications and credit that focus on occupational competence. Although the achievement of vocational credit within educational programmes can be used to meet the needs of purchasers in ensuring that staff are 'fit for purpose', it is essential that the requirements of statutory and professional bodies are also met within the programmes.

In the UK this approach is becoming more common in the professional domain, as reported in *The Future Health Care Workforce*: 'The professional bodies are increasingly aware of the need to deliver occupational competence. The Calman report on specialist medical training, for example, states that the completion of specialist medical training should be based on assessment of competence . . .' (Conroy 1996).

The UKCC have developed a framework of competences following the publication of *Fitness for Practice* (UKCC 1999a). These outcomes-based competences have been developed for entry to the branch programme, and for entry to the register. In the UK a number of universities are using the UKCC standards to adapt pre-registration programmes to enable students to be accredited with prior experience and learning. This process can result in students being given exemption from part of the first year of the pre-registration programme.

In order to demonstrate that they have met the standards, the practitioner must provide evidence of performance and evidence of capability (Eraut and Cole 1993). The former involves consideration of evidence obtained from the workplace whilst the latter focuses on the cognitive processes, concepts and theories that the practitioner has had to consider; in other words, the knowledge base which will supplement performance evidence (NBNI 2000).

Competence is not static; a healthcare professional can learn skills, but the knowledge underpinning a skill may change over time. This can affect the ability to practice the skill. In addition, practice is necessary to maintain competence (An Bord Altranais 2000a). The healthcare professional must acknowledge any limitations in competence and refuse in such cases to accept delegated or assigned functions. If appropriate, the professional must take appropriate measures to gain competence in the particular area. Competence is developmental and healthcare professionals must maintain competence and its continuing development through engaging in continuing professional development (UKCC 1992, An Bord Altranais 2000b).

Portfolios and lifelong learning

One method that is emerging for practitioners to demonstrate and record competence is the use of portfolios. Health professionals of all backgrounds are increasingly interested in applied learning which has a real-world validity and direct relevance to day-to-day practice. Portfolio building is an assessment system that is congruent with these aspirations. The portfolio system allows for closer integration of theory and practice. The portfolio system used in the Faculty of Health at the University of Central Lancashire has allowed for the closer integration of theory and practice. The competency-based outcome statements utilised within a number of our programmes avoid the perhaps false separation of theory from practice – a separation which may well have been fostered by the implied belief that it is indeed possible to divide the two. The thinking fostered by portfolio use has enabled lecturers to reconsider crucial curricular issues such as what to teach and how to teach it.

It has been found that students on programmes which use portfolios and competency-based outcome statements are, from the beginning, focused on their personal development in terms of direct vocational relevance. Additionally, the use of portfolios can enable the practitioner to subject their practice to scrutiny through reflective processes and experiential learning. Competency-based frameworks and the portfolio approach to assessment have the potential to bring together the best of both worlds (learning theories and learning on the job) through the development of programmes of learning which:

- assess theory through application in practice
- subject practice to scrutiny
- allow practitioners to reflect on the appropriateness of actions taken and alternatives to be considered.

The *Assessing Competencies in Nursing and Midwifery Education* project report (Bedford *et al.* 1993) includes a set of recommendations on practice assessment that promote the use of portfolios in assessment processes. These processes include several that match the requirements of an NVQ-type assessment.

- The assessment of clinical practice should require the collection of a range of forms of evidence to serve as the basis for student–assessor discussion about knowledge, skills, attitudes and understanding.
- The preparation of clinical area assessors should develop assessors' competence in collecting evidence, analysing data and developing frameworks for discussion.
- Assessment documentation should be broadened to include evidence contributed by more than one accredited witness.

Portfolios seem to be taking over the UK. Everywhere you turn these days you are being required to produce a portfolio of evidence. It starts at school, where all secondary pupils and some primary school pupils are issued with a National Record of Achievement that they start to compile before they are 11 years old, the principle behind this being that once they are conditioned and start portfolio building at an early age they will then continue to build portfolios for the rest of their lives (Storey 1996).

Portfolios are not only being used in secondary education. They are now being widely used in further and higher education for a variety of purposes. They are extensively used within the vocational qualification framework for NVQs and GNVQs as well as within many academic programmes at certificate, diploma and degree level. In many educational institutions portfolios are required for accreditation of prior learning

(APL). They can be used for two purposes; first for credit exemption from parts of a programme where the candidate demonstrates sufficient knowledge and experience for them to meet the learning outcomes, and secondly, for formal accreditation for units or modules towards an award such as a certificate, diploma or degree (Storey 1996).

However, the number of different competency frameworks that are emerging, the purposes for which they are to be used, and the way in which individuals present evidence that they are meeting the criteria identified in the frameworks are confusing the whole issue of competence.

To many people, portfolio production is like entering a strange land where you do not understand the language and the culture is different. Most people in the workforce these days have come through an education system that relies on testing of knowledge at the end of a period of learning, and therefore the production of portfolios for assessment presents them with riddles to solve and evidence to find.

Portfolios are not the easiest system for students and practitioners to master, however they do provide an effective mechanism to relate theory to practice. White (1994) claims that the portfolio system offers a view of student learning that is active, engaged and dynamic, as opposed to the overwhelming passivity that characterises other approaches to assessment, and can be a vehicle to bring teaching, learning and assessment together as mutually supportable activities (NBNI 2000).

The case against competency frameworks

Although there is a strong support for competence frameworks, there are critics of the process who suggest competency frameworks are reductionist, tend to be focused upon discrete tasks or behaviours, do not reflect the importance of the context in which practice takes place and do not portray the integrative, holistic nature of healthcare, i.e. that the whole is greater than the sum of its parts (WHO 2001). Jessup (1991), in his description of functional analysis, stated: 'The analysis and specification of competence according to functions, which is now advocated, provides a broader conception of competence than earlier task analysis approaches. The concentration on function shifts the focus of competence from tasks and procedures to the purpose and outcome of work activity.' The International Council of Nurses (2001) accept the criticisms and suggest that there is little doubt that frameworks are derived from the job/function or skill/task analysis of roles, but that there is some justification for developing detailed job-specific competencies.

There are a number of other arguments that can be made against the use of competency frameworks, especially within an NHS context.

- There is a danger that competency frameworks may be used to impose a training rather than an educational agenda.
- Competency-based approaches may not take account of individual aspirations and interests, which may have implications for retention and morale.
- At higher levels of expertise, characterised by the need for expertise and particularly the need to synthesise expertise from a range of domains, it may be difficult to define structured competencies.

Many of these issues can be exacerbated or ameliorated according to the manner of implementation. The competency set is a tool which may be used or misused. For this reason, in this book, we shall use a range of case studies to consider implementation issues.

2

Clinical governance and competent practitioners

The ability of organisations to provide effective, quality healthcare has been the subject of a number of policy and strategy documents within the NHS and independent sectors of healthcare. Clinical governance is seen as one strategy that will enable employers to subject their organisation to scrutiny and develop a competent workforce that meets customer and organisational needs.

Clinical governance has been defined as:

> A framework through which NHS organisations are accountable for continuously improving the quality of their services and safeguarding high standards of care by creating an environment in which excellence in clinical care will flourish.
>
> (DoH 1998a, b)

For clinical governance in primary care trusts, health authorities and acute trusts, new skills will be required throughout these organisations to deliver the improving standards of patient care which clinical governance entails. These include effective leadership, clinical audit, quality monitoring and improvement, but also a wide range of education and professional development initiatives that monitor and develop the competence of the workforce.

Nearly one million people work for the NHS. Two billion pounds a year is spent on supporting training and education for clinical staff – and more money is spent locally on staff development and training. 'We need to make sure that we plan and develop the NHS workforce, and use our investment in it to deliver the best, most effective, care for patients. Because caring for people is what the NHS is all about.' (DoH 2000b)

Good clinical governance is about saving money that would otherwise be spent on compensation for clinical negligence claims, investigations, etc. When the right system is not in place and staff do not have the appropriate competence to do their job, more money is spent to correct deficits, which leads to less money for patient care and fewer patients being treated through less resources being available to meet service needs.

The report *A Health Service of All the Talents* (DoH 2000b) stems from long-standing concerns about the way in which the NHS educates, trains and uses its staff. Its proposals and recommendations – which are summarised below – are wide-ranging and radical. But at their heart is a simple theme – that the NHS workforce, whose commitment no one can doubt, needs to be transformed in order to provide the sort of care that will be needed in the future. The emphasis needs to be on:

- *team working* across professional and organisational boundaries
- *flexible working* to make the best use of the range of skills and knowledge which staff have
- *streamlined workforce planning and development* which stems from the needs of patients, not of professionals
- *maximising the contribution of all staff to patient care*, doing away with barriers which say only doctors or nurses can provide particular types of care
- *modernising education and training* to ensure that staff are equipped with the skills they need to work in a complex, changing NHS
- *developing new, more flexible, careers* for staff of all professions
- *expanding the workforce* to meet future demands.

The report suggests that there is a need to do this not just because it is the right thing to do but because it will provide patients with the care they have the right to expect. Care which is delivered quickly, by skilled professionals who listen to them and provide the best possible treatment and care. The NHS has dedicated, hard-working but insufficient staff. The Government is committed to expanding the NHS by expanding the numbers of doctors, nurses and other health professionals. But alongside expansion must come reform, to change the way staff work, the way they are trained and how they are educated (DoH 2000b).

Employers need to maximise the skills of all their current staff and review the way in which jobs are designed and care delivered. There are a range of initiatives being undertaken by NHS trusts and other employers in this area – including the development of nurse consultant posts – but more needs to be done to drive this through the NHS and to ensure that the modernised pay systems proposed in *Agenda for Change* (NHS Executive 1999) are used to best effect. In developing and expanding the roles of health professionals it will be important not to lose staff's professional identities but to develop additional skills which will enable them to work more flexibly and give them more transferable skills. It will be important also to ensure that the skills and capabilities of staff are fully used. Decisions on who can provide care should start from the patient's needs, not professional background and training.

In one NHS trust, a review of policies and procedures in relation to equality and diversity reported 'the Trust, like any other similar employer, is fundamentally in the business of providing a high-quality healthcare service to meet patients' needs and requirements. It is the staff who will provide the services and the staff must be competent, skilful and experienced appropriately to do so' (BHRV NHS Trust 2000). They went on to suggest that 'having diverse staff from all backgrounds, who are competent in all aspects of the job that they are tasked to do, as well as being able to relate to patients of all backgrounds, will help to stimulate such trust and confidence thus enhancing the quality of services and improving overall performance' (BHRV NHS Trust 2000).

Competence and healthcare practitioners

The issue of the competence of practitioners is currently a key issue for healthcare providers. Recent inquiries, including the Bristol Royal Inquiry (NHS Executive 2001) and the inquiry into the Cardiac Unit in Oxford (NHS Executive 2000), have identified significant problems in relation to the continuing competence of healthcare practitioners.

The Bristol Inquiry noted that:

- there was no requirement on hospital consultants to keep their skills and knowledge up to date or to demonstrate to anyone other than their peer group that they remained sufficiently skilled
- the systems in existence were not capable of assuring the competence of healthcare professionals
- poor or diminishing competence could not be adequately addressed until it became manifestly bad.

The Bristol Inquiry argued that 'in the case of doctors and nurses, technical clinical skills are a necessary but not a sufficient qualification to practice as a healthcare professional. For the future we must expand our understanding of what constitutes professional competence. Attitudes and interpersonal skills must be recognised as having value alongside clinical skills. This has consequences for the way in which future healthcare professionals are selected and educated'(NHS Executive 2001).

In the twenty-first century, patients' expectations are greater than they have been in the past and they expect a professional service from professionals. As the Bristol Inquiry reported:

> Professional competence refers to patients' expectations that the professional they come into contact with will be up to the job. Professionals should be able to do that which they profess they can do. From the patient's point of view, it is shocking to think that this might not be the case.
>
> Indeed, the need for healthcare professionals to acquire and maintain appropriate levels of competence is so obvious that it would seem unnecessary to refer to it. The patient simply expects that the healthcare professional has up-to-date knowledge and skills. A healthcare professional's competence from the patient's point of view is not negotiable.
>
> (NHS Executive 2001)

In healthcare, as well as other professional areas, levels of competence vary because healthcare professionals have different experiences and different levels of knowledge. A consultant or a nurse ward manager will have a wider and deeper level of competence than the junior doctor or newly qualified nurse. Yet, even at the start of a professional life, competence should meet a critical minimum level.

In the past, graduation from a nursing programme and passage of licensure examinations was presumed to ensure competency of practitioners throughout their careers. Those days are indeed past and nursing has recently acknowledged that this is no longer realistic in today's practice arena with the rapid change in healthcare and explosion of nursing knowledge worldwide. Nurses must maintain competency in practice by updating their knowledge to assure quality care.

Professional competence requires a firm educational grounding, followed by a period of formal training to acquire the relevant knowledge and skills in the workplace. Thereafter, continued competence rests on a combination of education, continuous development, confidence and experience. It depends on the motivation of individual professionals to learn and develop and the extent to which their employer supports them and enables them to do so. It also depends on the professional standards which they are required or expected to meet, and on the wider systems for ensuring that those standards are adhered to. Thus, acquiring and maintaining professional competence involves collaboration between the individual, the educational institutions, the employer, and those who set and enforce standards of professional competence (NHS Executive 2001).

Individual healthcare professionals, once qualified, need to be sufficiently motivated and have sufficient incentive to maintain and develop their competence. If the process of keeping knowledge and skills up to date is neglected, the professional's level of competence will diminish (NHS Executive 2001).

As stated previously, competence can be seen as a continuum along which people can move. This can be backwards as well as forwards and it must be acknowledged that in any clinical situation competence can deteriorate if it is not maintained. Contexts change, new knowledge emerges and practice develops, therefore competence to practice needs to be redefined on a regular basis if the practitioner is to ensure that they are meeting the needs of their patients and the organisation.

Hogston (1993) reported that:

> Periodic registration will not itself guarantee that registered practitioners have maintained a level of competence.

If this is the case, then systems need to be in place to ensure that practitioners maintain their fitness for practice and fitness for purposes. The portfolio system can be utilised by the practitioner as a dynamic tool to demonstrate that competence is being maintained and developed over time. In a number of states in Australia, systematic auditing of a percentage of practitioners' professional portfolios has shown that:

- the majority of nurses are able to demonstrate continued competence
- a small number of nurses have left practice and not re-registered
- only two nurses required further education and professional development before they were reinstated to the register.

These formal processes appear to be having a significant impact on nurses, who have to subject their practice to scrutiny and ensure that they are competent to practice.

A knock-on effect of this auditing system is likely to be an increase in continuing professional development as a means for the registered nurse to update knowledge and practice. Auditing may also go some way to overcome the stagnation that was observed during my visit to some services in Australia, where staff had been in post for many years and had not undertaken any professional development – their practice had not changed during this time. The Australian audit system has some similarities to the pilot that the UKCC has undertaken to review selected portfolios when nurses seek to re-register with them (Storey 2001).

It is crucial, therefore, that the working life of healthcare professionals be so structured as to allow them to meet these requirements. This means that the employer must provide professionals with sufficient time and opportunity to maintain existing skills, and to acquire and consolidate new skills. Thus, the work environment in the NHS must support and enable the process of continuous learning through well-planned strategies for continuing professional development. As for those who set standards, they must ensure that their frameworks of professional standards are and remain appropriate to the needs of patients and professionals and are, in fact, observed.

Competency-based approaches and clinical governance

The competency-based approach to training and development is driven by employment-related performance objectives within the framework of the job description. This approach will provide an opportunity to facilitate continuing professional development that equates to the objectives of the organisation. Competency-based approaches allow clarity for managers and those responsible for both individual and institutional development regarding the connection between the role of the job and the skills required to deliver it. By developing and maintaining essential core competencies linked to tasks and responsibilities, the service places the development of the individual within the institution into context, and enables clear monitoring and qualitative testing (BHRV NHS Trust 2000). This means that the individual will not only be aware of what the job entails, through the job description, but also what they need to know and do in order to carry out their tasks efficiently, appropriately and efficiently, through occupational standards.

As the report to the Trust recommended, 'When incorporated into the management structure that incorporates essential personal and professional development, the requirement and design of training to support the competency framework can be directly related to service needs and output. The service's evaluation of its effective training would thus more easily be accomplished as it is directly related to the institutional imperatives in respect of competencies and diversity' (BHRV NHS Trust 2000).

The report identified that 'currently there is no core competency for staff, either for the specifics of race awareness, equal opportunities, diversity or other roles considered core to the employment within the service. Other organisations that have adopted core competencies as the basis of employment-related objectives have seen greater clarity of the role of their staff, training needs and any required management interventions' (BHRV NHS Trust 2000).

It is clear that the development of a competence framework pays benefits to healthcare organisations and enables them to develop a workforce that meets service needs and their obligations in relation to clinical governance. 'Current good practice is to develop core competencies, either as minimum effective training levels or occupational standards. The Trust may wish to follow this model . . . The competency framework would engage management, staff, their associations and all other interested parties to ensure effectiveness and guide their development. Its application informs management and the development of staff as well as designers and providers of training within the service' (BHRV NHS Trust 2000).

Development of competency frameworks

The development of competency frameworks relies on collaboration between key stakeholders, including employers, employees, service users, staff associations and education and training designers and providers. The framework design process includes functional analysis, which is a process that underpins the development of occupational standards. Functional analysis is a holistic, systems-based analysis approach used to analyse whole occupations in terms of outcomes and the purpose of work activities rather than specific activities, procedures and methods. This approach is used to facilitate the development of national occupational standards, which are presented in the form of a 'functional map'.

National occupational standards define the level of performance required for the successful achievement of work expectations. They specify best practice in an employment sector and are expressed in the form of elements of competence, performance criteria and range indicators. The range indicators are used as specifications for assessment when standards are aggregated together to form qualifications.

National Vocational Qualifications are qualifications based on standards developed through the process of functional analysis. NVQs are a selection of units of competence, taken from a set of occupational standards endorsed by the employment sector's lead body and which meet criteria laid down by the National Council for Vocational Qualifications.

Functional analysis gives educational providers a holistic view of the employment needs of an occupational area, and enables them to develop a curriculum that reflects these needs. The outcomes of functional analysis are a functional map, which outlines the key purpose, key areas and key roles that are required to provide a service to patients. A functional map is normally symbolised as a 'fallen tree' (as in Figure 2.1), which illustrates the stages of analysis and disaggregation that result in the development of occupational standards. Occupational standards are statements of competence, national specifications for performance, which include the ability to perform in a range of work-related activities. With the under-pinning skills, knowledge and understanding required, they describe what should happen in employment (NCVQ 1989, Mansfield and Mitchell 1996).

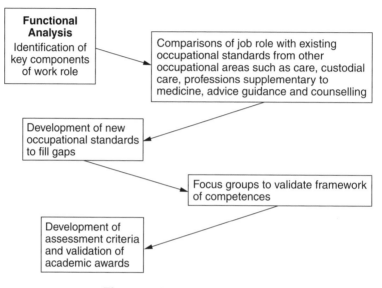

Figure 2.1   Functional map.

Functional analysis suffers from inappropriate links to 'functionalism', a 1960s approach to the description and analysis of social action. It also suffers from claims of 'reductionism, mechanistic, conforming, resistant to change and deterministic' (Mansfield and Mitchell 1996, p. 99) which stem from the analytical approach used in order to determine occupational standards.

Mansfield and Mitchell (1996, p. 101) report that functional analysis has its origins in the hermeneutic and dialectical traditions of social science, relating to the social theories and methodologies of interpret-ative understanding which reject the reductionist and behaviourist approaches which attempted to define and analyse social action using empirical methods adopted by the natural sciences. They go on to say that functional analysis was developed 'for the sole purpose of developing descriptions of human capability . . . by concentrating on the expectations of employment, broken down through a process of structured analysis which eventually produces a level of detail which we describe as an occupational standard' (Mansfield and Mitchell 1996, p. 101).

Functional analysis – the process

Functional analysis determines the key purpose of an occupational area through consultation with the job holders (experts). The analysis identifies current best practices and balances these against realistic future expectations. The key purpose and key roles of the occupation are determined by asking practitioners simple, but searching, questions, such as:

- What are you seeking to achieve?
- What are the expected outcomes of your work?
- What are the values that underpin and tensions that impinge on your delivery of care?

From the responses, analysts are able to produce a 'map' of the occupational area, which includes key purpose and key roles. Key roles are then broken up into sub-sets of units made up of performance standards. It is this process of breaking up or disaggregating a role which alarms many educationalists. Dymott (1994) supports this view by stating that NVQs could result in nursing becoming a de-skilled and mechanistic profession. However, Oakes (1994), Eaton (1994), Storey *et al.* (1995a, b) and Mansfield and Mitchell (1996) argue that the adoption and the use of occupational standards does not necessarily lead to task orientation (or mechanistic practice).

Wolf (1994, p. 3) points out that the process of defining standards in terms of units, elements, performance criteria and range statements means that what is integrated is, in reality, often disaggregated in the assessment specification for an NVQ. However, as Mansfield and Mitchell (1996, p. 127) point out, it is important to keep occupational standards and NVQs separate. NVQs are but one of the ways in which occupational standards may be used. They can also be used to define job descriptions; to provide a benchmark for individual and organisational development; as a means of assessment of performance; as a tool for training needs analysis; and to form qualifications.

Specificity of standards

A contentious issue in discussions about standards concerns the optimum level of specificity. If there is too little specificity, the result may be a lack of clarity, poor communication and diminished credibility. On the other hand, too much specificity can lead to standards which take too long to read, are cumbersome and can lead to abuse of the system by people taking short cuts. This criticism has been directed at the national occupational standards from certain occupational areas, although it is accepted that different parts of the same set of occupational standards may require different levels of specificity (Eraut and Cole 1993, Beaumont 1996, CBI 1994).

If one role of standards is to establish a reasonable level of agreement and common understanding about the definition of competence, it is true that well-defined standards will do this more effectively than poorly defined standards. It must be recognised, though, that there are limits to what written standards can achieve on their own. Total uniformity of interpretation is an unattainable goal.

The formulation of standards involves a great deal of professional judgement. The variations in work role and working practice between one job and another, within an occupational area, can be quite large. It is important that standards are based on a thorough analysis of the nature of professional work and its knowledge base. There should also be an assumption that some capacity for change should be built into the standards themselves in order to ensure that students and professionals are not judged by out-of-date criteria, and that there is a clear statement of the methodology and rationale used to derive the standards, which should be documented in an explicit way (Eraut and Cole 1993, p. 25). Functional analysis does this, in that the outcome of the analysis is a functional map which outlines the key purpose, key roles and functions of the occupational area.

Educating the future workforce

It is accepted that a skilled and knowledgeable workforce is essential to achieving many of the strategic objectives highlighted by a variety of policy documents, and reports, including *The NHS Plan* (DoH 2000a), *A Health Service of All the Talents* (DoH 2000b) and the National Service Frameworks that are emerging for specific areas of care, including cancer care and mental health.

Education and training for healthcare professionals has to take account of these and future policy changes if they wish to produce the competent and relevantly educated practitioners of the future. It is essential that the products of faculties and departments in higher education are viewed as 'fit for purpose', whilst also perceived as providing 'value for money'.

This view was originally highlighted by the Department of Health (1994) in its 'Statement of Strategic Intent' for the nursing, midwifery and health-visiting professions, and in recent Executive Letters, for example EL(95)96, where they advocate the use of occupational standards in educational programmes, and has been supported more recently in the UKCC's *Fitness for Practice* (1999a) and the Department of Health's *Making a Difference* (1999) documents.

Occupational standards and professional development

Approaches to the integration of occupational standards within higher education have been attempted in a number of institutions. The conference proceedings from the Universities Association for Continuing Education (1996) recorded a number of initiatives where occupational standards and traditional higher education processes are being merged. One paper in particular (Parker 1996, p. 39) reflected on experiences of using NVQs in higher education and the comparability between professional curricula in higher education and NVQs. In spite of inherent differences between the models, several ways of integrating the two approaches were suggested. These included:

- the incorporation of NVQ units accredited within HE curricula – this would involve linking pure knowledge (HE focus) with competence (NVQ focus) by assessing understanding in the workplace
- the development of portfolios of NVQs at levels 4 and 5 after obtaining a university certificate or diploma
- recognition that management lends itself to NVQ awards, but that there are difficulties with other disciplines
- and that progression can be built into NVQ achievement, but only in terms of closing the gap between an individual's present and desired future performance (Parker 1996, p. 39).

3

The model

Introduction: the context

In the six months prior to the writing of this book, the rationale for using competency-based training tools was highlighted on a number of occasions. This was not just by the publication of various reports, discussed earlier, but on a personal level, in discussions with a number of senior individuals with remits for education and training within the National Health Service. The remarks that were made on several occasions were along the lines of: 'I can't afford to do a training needs analysis because I haven't got the money to fund the training that would be identified.' Or 'I haven't got time to do a training needs analysis, the money has to be spent before April.' From an outside perspective this appears somewhat confusing, if not perverse, when placed in the context of the training budgets under consideration, in each case extending well into six figures.

So on what basis do managers within the National Health Service identify the education and training needs of the staff that they are responsible for? The annual appraisal meeting with a manager would go something like this:

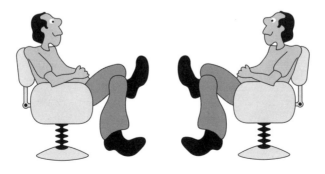

> *Manager*: So here we are again.
> *Me*: Yes, here we are again.
> *Manager*: So, when did you last do a course?
> *Me*: Ooh, about a year ago.
> *Manager*: Want to do another one?
> *Me*: OK.
> *Manager*: What course do you fancy?
> *Me*: How about that one the University keep going on about, I haven't done that one yet.
> *Manager*: OK, sign here and I'll see you next year.

Obviously, this may be a slight exaggeration, but from experience, training needs assessment is virtually universally bottom up and consists of the simple question: what would you like to do next? If there is enough money left in the budget and it is your turn, then you get to go on your chosen course. The obvious exception to this is in the area of mandatory training, which will be discussed shortly.

The effect of this approach to education and training is to allow some individuals to wander the corridors of academia, collecting qualifications in the same way they do the weekly shop at the supermarket.

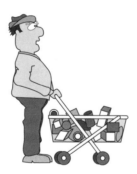

These courses and qualifications may have little, if any, relationship to what is actually needed in order to assist them to do the job they are employed to do. Others, if they keep quiet and manage to avoid their manager's gaze, may undertake only the bare minimum of mandatory training. More importantly, there is no analysis of the skills or knowledge which staff already possess or exploration of the skills and knowledge they need, both now and in the future.

So what about the notion of mandatory training? All staff in the health service are required to attend a fire-safety lecture once a year. The important point here is attendance. This mandatory training owes little to theories of education or acquisition and retention of skills and knowledge but much to litigation prevention and possibly even to be seen to be 'doing something about it'. To a lesser extent this also occurs with resuscitation training, although here at least there is an opportunity to practise clinical skills.

With this in mind, and on the basis of several years' work, we set about the task of finding a better way – possibly not the holy grail or the answer to life, the universe and everything, but at least a rational framework upon which both managers and clinicians may base their assessment of current situations and the skills and knowledge development needed to deliver the service in the future.

Development of a model

One of the major changes currently facing the NHS is the introduction of the electronic health record and the electronic patient record. These developments obviously bring with them new technology, which leads to new skill requirements for staff. Even the most expensive, hi-tech, top-of-the-range patient record system is simply a heap of plastic and metal boxes in the corner collecting dust unless someone knows how to switch it on. It remains fairly useless if the appropriate staff do not know how to use key functions, and only when the operators are skilled enough to actually utilise all of the electronic wizardry does the heap in the corner begin to become an asset rather than a liability.

So how do we go about ensuring staff have the appropriate skills they need? Obviously, we need to decide what skills are needed and then measure individual performance against these. Bentley (1996) outlines two paradigms for performance. Firstly, what might be called the traditional competency-based approach, that is, a measurement of how well people are doing the things that they do with little regard to the eventual outcome ('the operation was a success but the patient died'), and secondly, by disregarding the way in which things are done and simply looking at the outcomes ('never mind the quality, feel the width'). This is the output-focused approach to performance management.

The authors have attempted to bridge this paradigm divide by using a model that includes competencies as well as an element of outcome. A fundamental problem with the Benner model described earlier is that, across the board, an individual's performance is not necessarily uniform across all aspects of their role. Performance in various areas of practice may be at different levels, depending on background knowledge and previous experience. The development of the model described in Chapter

5 is thus our preferred rating scale of performance. However, the flexibility of the model is such that any performance-rating scale may be used.

As a starting point we took a competency framework developed within what was then the College of Nursing and Health Studies, later to evolve into the Faculty of Health, and stripped out the competencies to leave the basic framework. For those of you with an anorak, the model at this point looks exactly like a spreadsheet. For those of you only slightly further down the evolutionary ladder, it looks like a chessboard. For everyone else, it looks like a draughtboard.

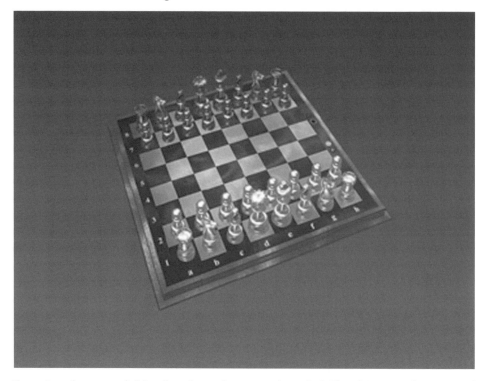

Imagine the top of this chessboard as a series of skills, things to know and ways of behaving, with each line of squares taken up for one individual skill, thing or behaviour. Along the other side of our board we have all different sorts of people. People who do the same sort of job would form an orderly queue to the side of one line of squares.

If we now look at our chessboard, we see a series of columns (the lines of squares going up and down), each representing an individual skill, bit of knowledge, or behaviour. Along the other edge of the board we have a series of rows (the line of squares going from side to side), each representing a different 'sort' of person or a different 'role' which they perform.

So for me as an individual, when I find the right queue to stand in, in front of me will be a series of squares, each one representing a skill, bit of knowledge, etc. Imagine that instead of a chess piece in each of these squares is a one of those old 'test your strength' machines that used to be found in travelling fairgrounds. They consist of a big button and an even bigger hammer that you had to hit as hard as you could, the aim being to see how far up the scale you could push the little marker. Only on this scale are not the usual 'Weed', 'Weakling', 'Muscle Man', 'Super Hero', etc. but a level set by a group of experts which tells me how high I should be able to get the marker in that particular square. If I then test my skill in that particular square I can tell a couple of things. Not just my absolute level of skill, strength or even weakness, as measured by how far up I can push the marker, but I will clearly see whether this is at, above or below the level which I should be in that square.

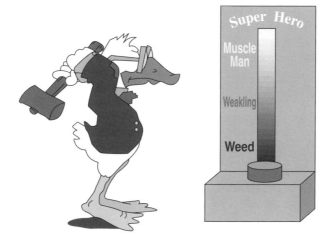

If we now try to look at our chessboard analogy in a little more detail, it becomes clear that this is fine just as long as there is only one person wanting to use each row of the board. In the same way that when playing chess each square has room for only one piece at a time, each square of our matrix can only hold information about one person at a time.

The obvious answer is to give each player their own row of squares, but there are a number of drawbacks to this in terms of designing an integrated system, as although this approach would allow the individual to see their own development needs, analysing all of these individual matrices is more than a little difficult.

What we really need to do is to transform our model from a chessboard into a database. We will pause here whilst those of you who struggled with the idea of a spreadsheet go for a little lie down somewhere.

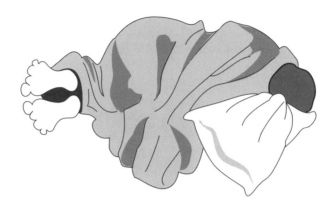

Feel better now? Then on we go. Don't worry, as we won't go into huge detail, but essentially what we have done is to take this chessboard and turn it into a virtual chessboard. Computers, being very clever, do not need to draw a row of squares for every person who might ever be going to use our matrix. Instead, we simply tell the computer what the board looks like, what roles and what competency items there are and finally what the minimum acceptable level is in each square. Then the computer can make a copy of the appropriate row for each user to use as the need arises.

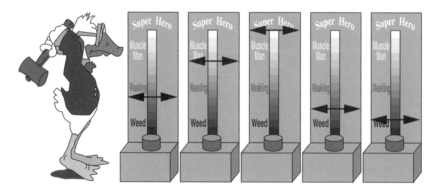

Now each user, as far as they are concerned, has their own row of squares with the scale on the machine in each square set to where it should be for their role in that competency item.

In order to decide whether or not you have a training need in a particular area, all you need to do is to visit each square along your row and 'test your strength' against the level that you should be able to achieve in that item. In this way the system can build up a profile of the actual skill or performance level you possess in relation to each item and also the gap between your performance and that required by your role. Education and training can then be based on developing the skills you actually need to do your job.

4

Case study 1:
Developing competency-based frameworks for nurses within Blackburn, Hyndburn & Ribble Valley NHS Trust

Introduction

This initiative emerged as a consequence of the report of the review of the Trust's strategies, policies, practices and processes on racial equality (BHRV NHS Trust 2000) and the development and implementation of their Nursing and Midwifery Strategy (BHRV NHS Trust 2001). Both of these documents advocated the development of a competency framework in order to develop the skills of the Trust's workforce and to enable it to develop effective training and development strategies.

The review of equality and ethnicity concluded that 'there is no core competency for staff, either for the specifics of race awareness, equal opportunities, diversity or other roles considered core to employment within the service. Other organisations that have adopted core competencies as the basis of employment-related objectives have seen greater clarity of the role of their staff, training needs and any required management interventions' (BHRV NHS Trust 2000).

The report also suggested that current good practice is to develop core competencies, either as minimum effective training levels or as occupational standards. 'The competency framework would engage management, staff and their associations and all other interested parties to ensure effectiveness and guide their development. Its application informs personal and professional development, management and the development of staff, as well as the designers and providers of training within the service' (BHRV NHS Trust 2000).

The Trust, within its *Nursing and Midwifery Strategy 2001–2004* (BHRV NHS Trust 2001), also recognised a requirement to develop competency frameworks linked to job descriptions for nurses across a range of grades, including healthcare assistants, and nurses at D, E, F and G grades from Medicine, Surgery, Critical Care, A&E (excluding theatre staff), Elderly, Obstetrics and Gynaecology.

The Director of Personnel & Development, Blackburn, Hyndburn & Ribble Valley NHS Trust commissioned the resulting project. The project team consisted of two senior lecturers from the Faculty of Health, University of Central Lancashire and an experienced Human Resources and Training Manager from another trust, all of whom participated in the project on a sessional basis.

Background to competency frameworks

For the purpose of the project the following definitions were used:

- 'Competencies' are the knowledge, skills, abilities and behaviours that an employee applies in performing his/her work and are the key employee-related levers for achieving results that are relevant to the organisation's business strategies.
- A 'competency framework' is a set of competencies and includes associated behaviours that link directly to overall strategic priorities and the work that needs to be done to achieve them, as well as to levels of proficiency for each behaviour. The framework provides the proficiency levels and behaviours required for a specific job or jobs.

A competency framework applies to a specific employee or population of employees. It can cover employees in a group of positions/jobs within a department, or employees belonging to a functional community.

Frameworks can be applied in order to:

- recruit and select new staff
- monitor and evaluate individual and team performance (using 360-degree feedback)
- identify specific training and development needs
- develop training programmes to meet organisational, individual and team needs.

Proposed implementation plan to develop competency frameworks

The initiative was to be delivered over a number of phases that were evaluated and amended at each stage:

- Phase 1 – Pre-development meeting
- Phase 2 – Prepare an implementation plan for the project
- Phase 3 – Trust to request participation of nurses in the interview stage
- Phase 4 – Individual interviews
- Phase 5 – Analyse results and prepare draft competency frameworks
- Phase 6 – Focus groups to refine draft frameworks
- Phase 7 – Presentation of the competency frameworks and proposed implementation plan.

Phase 1 – Pre-development meeting

The pre-development meeting was scheduled between key personnel from the Trust and the faculty team. The purpose of the meeting was to:

- carry out a complete requirements analysis, so that all parties could be in agreement as to the outcomes of the programme
- define the groups and levels of staff that would be involved
- establish sample groups.

Phase 2 – Prepare an implementation plan for the project

A draft implementation plan was developed that identified the key:

- stages
- stakeholders
- timescales
- processes to be applied
- milestones to be achieved.

This draft plan was subject to agreement between the Trust and the project team at the university.

At this stage of the process, a draft competency framework and proficiency ladder were developed. The competency framework was developed from a range of sources. Over the last few years a number of competency frameworks have been developed, including those associated with National Vocational Qualifications (Care Sector Consortium 1989), standards for pre-registration nursing (UKCC 1999a), Liverpool University Hospitals NHS Trust (O'Hanlon and Andrews 1997), standards for a higher level of practice (UKCC 1999b) and competence for staff working with personality-disordered patients (Storey *et al*. 1997). This framework of competences was supplemented by a proficiency ladder that attempted to identify the appropriate levels of competence that were needed by staff at different grades throughout the Trust.

The proficiency ladder implemented in the Trust was adapted from Benner's novice to expert model (Benner 1984) in which she identified five levels of practice. Benner's model was based on the Dreyfus model (Dreyfus and Dreyfus 1980). The Dreyfus model identified five levels of proficiency:

- novice
- advanced beginner
- competent
- proficient
- expert.

Benner used this model to define levels of practice in nursing. She defined the levels as follows.

- **Novice:** That stage in the Dreyfus model of skill acquisition where no background understanding of the situation exists, so that context-free rules and attributes are required for safe entry and performance in the situation. It is unusual for a graduate nurse to be a novice, but it is possible. For example, an expert nurse in gerontology would be a novice in a neonatal intensive care unit. Many first year nursing students will begin at the novice stage; however, students who have had experience as nursing assistants will not be novice in basic nursing skills.
- **Advanced beginner:** One who can demonstrate marginally acceptable performance; one who has coped with enough real situations to note, or to have pointed out by a mentor, recurring meaningful situational components. The advanced beginner has enough background experience to recognise aspects of a situation.
- **Proficient:** The proficient performer perceives situations as wholes rather than in terms of aspects, and performance is guided by maxims. There is a qualitative leap or discontinuity in problem approach between the proficient and competent level of performance. The proficient performer recognises a situation in terms of overall picture. This person recognises which aspects of the situation are most salient. The proficient performer has an intuitive grasp of the situation based upon a deep background understanding.

- **Competent:** A stage in the Dreyfus model of skill acquisition typified by considerable conscious, deliberate planning. The plan indicates which attributes and aspects of the current and contemplated future situation are to be considered most important and which can be ignored. The competent stage is evidenced by an increased level of efficiency.
- **Expert:** Developed only when the clinician tests and refines theoretical and practical knowledge in actual clinical situations. Expertise develops through a process of comparing whole similar and dissimilar clinical situations with one another, so an expert has a deep background understanding of clinical situations based upon many past paradigm cases. Expertise is a hybrid of practical and theoretical knowledge.

Although the Benner model provided a basis for developing a proficiency ladder, it was felt that the definitions did not provide clear specifications for roles or grades, therefore a simplified version of the model was developed. In the proficiency ladder we attempted to define levels of responsibility and accountability that would be associated with each of the competency statements. Within the Trust it was acknowledged that for each of the competency items in the competency framework, the levels of attainment may vary from ward to ward or department and will also vary across and between the different grades. Therefore it was important to have definitions of levels that could be used to analyse job roles and responsibilities and then to determine individual practitioners' current position in relation to the agreed proficiency levels.

It was also accepted that competence is not static, therefore it was decided to label the levels as follows:

- foundation
- intermediate
- proficient
- advanced
- expert.

The following descriptions identify the potential level of attainment for nurses and healthcare assistants within the Trust. The levels can apply to HCAs or registered nurses dependent on their role and responsibility within their area of practice. In some circumstances registered nurses may be required to attain level 3 or 4 whilst in others they may only practice at levels 1 or 2.

For the purpose of this document 'practitioner' refers to all staff involved in care delivery.

Table 4.1 Proficiency levels.

Level	Description
Level 0	This does not form a part of the current or future role of the worker.
Level 1 – Foundation	The practitioner would contribute to care delivery whilst under the direct supervision of others more proficient in this competency. (This level of attainment may apply to the practitioner gaining experience and developing skills and knowledge in the competency.)
Level 2 – Intermediate	The practitioner can demonstrate acceptable performance in the competency and has coped with enough real situations in the workplace to require less supervision and guidance, but they are not expected to demonstrate full competence or practice autonomously.
Level 3 – Proficient	A practitioner who consistently applies the competency standard. The practitioner demonstrates competence through the skills and ability to practice safely and effectively without the need for direct supervision. (The proficient practitioner may practice autonomously, and supervise others, within a restricted range of competences.)
Level 4 – Advanced	The advanced practitioner is autonomous and reflexive, perceives situations as wholes, delivers care safely and accurately and is aware of current best practice. Advanced practitioners understand a situation as a whole because they perceive its meaning in terms of long-term goals. (The advanced practitioner is likely to be leading a team, delivering and supervising care delivery, evaluating the effectiveness of care being delivered and may also contribute to the education and training of others.)
Level 5 – Expert	The expert practitioner is able to demonstrate a deeper understanding of the situation and contributes to the development and dissemination of knowledge through the teaching and development of others. The expert practitioner is likely to have their own caseload and provide advice, guidance and leadership to other professionals involved in the delivery or provision of health and social care.

Phase 3 – Trust to request participation of nurses in the interview stage

A sample of nurses representing the range of grades was requested to participate in validating the draft competency framework. Their involvement took the form of participating in a one-to-one interview and completing the job analysis/proficiency level questionnaire.

Phase 4 – Individual interviews

Interviews were approximately 45 minutes in duration and focused on the role and responsibilities perceived to be inherent in the post holder's current post. The interviewers used a diagnostic job analysis and proficiency level questionnaire designed around the job descriptions.

Interviews were also undertaken with a number of the post holders' line managers to establish a comparison between expectations of line managers and the perceptions of post holders.

Managers from ten directorates within the Trust submitted their responses to the job analysis/proficiency level questionnaires. These responses were collated for analysis and it became apparent that there were significant variances in managers' expectations of the roles of post holders, as can be seen from the following example for A-grade competencies.

Table 4.2 Variances in managers' responses.

Competency	Directorate 1	Directorate 2	Directorate 3	Directorate 4	Directorate 5
Maintain the trust and support of colleagues and team members	1	2	1	3	3
Maintain the trust and support of one's immediate manager	1	3	1	3	3
Minimise interpersonal conflict	1	2	1	3	3
Help team members who have problems effecting their performance	1	0	1	2	0
Contribute to informal meetings and group discussions	1	2	1	2	3

Phase 5 – Analyse results and prepare draft competency frameworks

The data generated from the interviews was collated for cluster analysis to determine the generic competencies that would make up:

- the different competency frameworks for the varying roles
- those core generic competencies based on the overall picture across all nurse groups and levels
- proficiency levels for each grade across the framework of competencies.

This was achieved through convening a group of managers to reach a consensus on the baseline competences and proficiency levels for each grade from A through to G. It was acknowledged that in some areas nurses at different grades would need to perform above the baseline in order to deliver the service.

Phase 6 – Focus groups to refine draft frameworks

A series of focus groups involving a sample of senior nurses were held. The purpose of the focus groups was:

- to provide an opportunity for a wider range of staff to contribute to the consultation and have ownership of the process
- to further refine the competency frameworks
- to validate or identify deficiencies in the draft frameworks
- to identify contextual differences between different levels of nursing staff and in different work areas
- to reach consensus on the minimum proficiency level for each grade of staff across the trust.

It is interesting to note that in areas of the framework relating to 'basic nursing care' it was agreed that the same level of proficiency was required.

Table 4.3 'Basic care competencies' needing common levels of proficiency.

Competency	A Grade	B Grade	C Grade	D Grade	E Grade	F Grade	G Grade
Enable clients to maintain their personal cleanliness	3	3	3	3	3	4	4
Support clients in personal grooming and dressing	3	3	3	3	3	4	4
Assist in the transfer of a deceased person to an agreed location	2	2	3	3	4	4	4
Help clients to get ready for eating and drinking	3	3	3	3	3	4	4
Help clients to consume food and drink	3	3	3	3	3	4	4
Help clients to choose food and drink	3	3	3	3	4	4	5
Prepare and serve food and drink to clients	3	3	3	3	3	4	4

Whilst in other areas it is clear that there is a need to increase proficiency as nurses move through the grading structure.

Table 4.4 Competencies requiring increasing proficiency.

Competency	A Grade	B Grade	C Grade	D Grade	E Grade	F Grade	G Grade
Store and retrieve records	1	2	2	2	3	4	4
Collect and evaluate feedback to assess for wider applications	0	1	2	2	3	4	4
Make recommendations for clinically effective practice	0	1	2	3	3	4	5
Identify opportunities for improvement in services products and systems	1	1	3	3	4	4	5
Evaluate proposed changes for benefits and disadvantages	1	1	3	3	4	4	5
Negotiate and agree the introduction to change	1	1	2	3	3	4	5
Implement and evaluate changes to services products and systems	1	2	2	3	3	4	5

Phase 7 – Presentation of the competency frameworks and proposed implementation plan

The frameworks were presented to key personnel, along with recommendations for their implementation, to identify training needs, develop personal development plans and thus arrive at a strategic training plan.

Success criteria

It was of paramount importance to the success of the programme that:

- the commitment of managers was felt and believed throughout the organisation
- staff were fully aware of the benefits of competency frameworks to the individual and the organisation
- staff were fully briefed on the logistics of the process
- staff were aware that participation was not compulsory
- support and guidance were given to those participating in the interviews and focus groups
- a communication plan was in place to support the development and implementation of the competence framework.

5

Case study 2:
Staff development amongst staff assessing and treating personality disorder

Introduction

This case study is included to show how competency frameworks have been applied in practice. The area of personality disorder shares with other specialist disciplines a need for specialist skills not provided within a general pre-registration education and training. The case study describes the background and processes used to apply competence frameworks in this environment.

Unlike the other case studies, this study does not utilise the 'proficiency ladder' approach described in the previous chapter. However, a number of academic awards have been developed from the framework. These awards use the same competency statements but are assessed using different academic criteria to differentiate between the different roles and responsibilities undertaken by the diverse range of disciplines participating in the education and training programmes.

Background

Over recent years the needs of people with a personality disorder have been identified as being significantly different to those of people with a mental illness. However, the pre-registration education and training of professionals in the United Kingdom appears to be deficient (Storey *et al.* 1995a, b), particularly in relation to patients with a personality disorder. Organisations providing care for these people are having to develop or purchase education and training to fill the gaps. Ashworth Hospital Authority, near Liverpool, is one such organisation.

Ashworth Hospital Authority and the Faculty of Health, University of Central Lancashire are attempting to remedy this problem through the development of a framework of professional occupational standards that will ensure quality provision of care for people with a personality disorder. The High Security Psychiatric Services Commissioning Board, in the UK, has acknowledged these problems and supported this research in an attempt to address these issues.

The patient group who will benefit from this development has specific needs and is also subject to rigorous security requirements. The National Health Service Act 1977 (Section 4) requires the Secretary of State to provide special hospitals for detained mentally disordered patients 'who in his opinion require treatment under conditions of special security on account of their dangerous, violent or criminal propensities'. Ashworth Hospital is one of three such hospitals serving England and Wales which provides conditions of special security and draws its patients from the north of England, Wales, West Midlands and the London area.

When considering an application for a placement of a patient in Ashworth Hospital, there are three main issues which need to be considered:

1   the presence or absence of a recognisable mental disorder, i.e. mental illness, psychopathic disorder, mental impairment or severe mental impairment and any other disorder or disability of mind. It is psychopathic disorder (now more correctly referred to as the clinical condition of personality disorder) that this work and paper addresses
2   whether that individual presents as a grave and immediate danger to the public
3   whether (in relation to severe mental impairment, mental impairment or psychopathic disorder) that person will be amenable to treatment.

Personality disorder

In the last ten years, interest in personality disorder research has shown substantial growth. Personality disorders were, no doubt, catapulted into a prominent position by the creation of a special axis, axis 2, with its release in the third edition of the *Diagnostic and Statistical Manual on Mental Disorders* (DSM III) (American Psychiatric Association 1980). Research interest in personality disorders can be documented by the fact that over 750 empirical studies are abstracted in the American Psychological Association Psyc-lit database, covering the five year period of January 1987 to June 1992. The *Journal of Personality Disorders* is devoted exclusively to this area. The many national and international conferences and workshops that have been held on personality disorders are also a test to this growth.

This large and growing literature on personality disorders should not obscure the fact that there are serious theoretical and methodological problems with the whole personality disorder diagnostic enterprise. Indeed, the last rigorous evaluation of the diagnosis and treatment efficacy for this patient group, carried out by one of the Read subgroups in 1992 (Dolan and Coid 1992), outlined the major problems and disagreements amongst clinicians about the diagnosis of this condition and, if diagnosis was agreed, whether in fact the condition was amenable to treatment.

The whole subject area surrounding personality disorder was the subject of scrutiny with the publication of *The Mask of Sanity* (Cleckley 1976). This was used by Hare to develop a personality disorder diagnostic assessment tool. The tool comprised of items structured around descriptions of characteristics central to the diagnosis of psychopathy (Hare 1980, Hare *et al.* 1990), which has now become the formal assessment system known as the Revised Psychopathy Checklist:

Table 5.1 Revised Psychopathy Checklist.

Characteristics		Not present	Partially present	Fully present
		0	1	2
I.	Glibness/superficial charm			
II.	Grandiose sense of self-worth			
III.	Need for stimulation/proneness to boredom			
IV.	Pathological lying			
V.	Conning/manipulative			
VI.	Lack of remorse or guilt			
VII.	Shallow affect			
VIII.	Callous/lack of empathy			
IX.	Parasitic lifestyle			
X.	Poor behavioural controls			
XI.	Promiscuous sexual behaviour			
XII.	Early behaviour problems			
XIII.	Lack of realistic long-term goals			
XIV.	Impulsivity			
XV.	Irresponsibility			
XVI.	Failure to accept responsibility for actions			
XVII.	Many short-term marital relationships			
XVIII.	Juvenile delinquency			
XIX.	Revocation of conditional release			
XX.	Criminal versatility			

The checklist is scored on a simple 0, 1, 2 rating depending on whether this characteristic is not present, whether it is partially present or whether the condition is fully met. A scoring of 30+ is required for a diagnosis of psychopathy. The people who present with these personality traits are not only difficult to diagnose and difficult to treat, but from a nursing perspective provide extreme challenges in being able to provide care for.

Ashworth Hospital re-organisation

In December 1993, Ashworth Hospital Authority re-organised its internal clinical services and formed four clinical units. Two units focused on the needs of people with mental health problems, one unit was concerned with people who presented with special needs, including women patients, the elderly and people with a learning disability, and the fourth unit met the needs of people with a personality disorder.

This was the first time that people with the condition of personality disorder had been brought together in large numbers and dealt with as a single treatment entity. The unit comprises six wards catering for 130 patients and is the single largest unit for personality disorder within western Europe. In its evaluation of Ashworth Hospital services in 1994, the Health Advisory Services commended Ashworth Hospital for its decision to focus on this group.

Over the past two years the organisation has learnt experientially from the difficulties involved with this new venture in the development and delivery of care to this particularly challenging group.

An evident issue was the fact that people who had received nurse training within mental health, be they registered mental nurses or registered nurses for the mentally handicapped (nowadays referred to as patients with a learning disability), had had little or no preparation for working with a group with a primary diagnosis of personality disorder. The curricula for these forms of training often paid scant attention to this diagnostic area. In clinical placements, if professionals came into contact with personality disorders, it tended to be as a secondary diagnosis rather than a primary one. Indeed, it must be noted that as a primary diagnostic feature, this group is only met in any level of concentration in special hospitals, the prison service and in smaller numbers in the regional secure units. It was very evident, therefore, that any training for staff in relation to this group would need to be home-grown, drawing on the experience of people who had worked with this group and in this environment.

Whilst examination of the available research material describing this patient group is helpful, there is very little evidence regarding the nursing care or therapeutic milieu. The hospital decided therefore to take an ambitious and systematic decision to address this training shortfall and deficiency.

The hospital was eager to contribute to the development of a curriculum that was based on competences. In discussion with colleagues from the Faculty of Health, University of Central Lancashire, it was decided to investigate the possibility of developing a framework of standards for professional practice that was based on the methodology used to develop national occupational standards. It was felt that using this methodology would result in the development of a curriculum that would enable the identification of training needs and the recognition of an individual's current abilities.

National occupational standards

National occupational standards are descriptions or benchmarks against which an individual's performance can be judged. In a study by Eraut and Cole (1993) it was stated that all professions should have public statements about what their qualified members are competent to do and what can reasonably be expected from them. These should comprise both minimum occupational standards and codes of professional conduct. The public statements could also include information about more specialist services provided by those with additional expertise and/or further qualifications. It was felt that, whilst most of the requirements of a code of conduct should be embedded within occupational standards, it was nevertheless important to have a separate statement of the ethical foundations of the work of a profession and the commitments made by its members.

It follows therefore that national occupational standards can be used by professions:

1   to inform the public and employers about the claims to competence of the profession. This is an essential starting point for any discussions about the role of the profession;
2   to inform the public and employers about the strength of its quality assurance systems so that individual clients can have clear expectations of the service to be provided;
3   to inform those who provide professional education and training about the goals to be achieved by students for entry to the profession;

4 where appropriate, they may be incorporated into regulations or criteria for the approval of courses and/or practice settings;

5 to provide guidance for students, placement supervisors and teachers about the competences students are expected to achieve;

6 to provide a foundation for the design of valid and reliable assessment systems for qualifications;

7 to establish European equivalencies and/or criteria for granting professional status in the United Kingdom to nurses who have trained and practised abroad.

(Eraut and Cole 1993)

The potential of National Vocational Qualifications (NVQs)/national occupational standards in higher education has already been recognised by a number of institutions; for example, the Vocational Qualifications Unit of the Open University has gone through considerable expansion and is involved in the development of learning systems to support workplace assessment and learning. In addition, it has been involved in the identification of guidance pathways for those individuals who wish to achieve both vocational accreditation from an NVQ assessment centre and academic accreditation from the Open University.

Stephenson (1993) argues that an integration of knowledge and skills within the curriculum (through the medium of workplace assessment) provides a coherent and relevant experience for the student. Eraut and Cole (1993) point out, however, that the workplace-based training element of professional preparation within higher education (HE) programmes is often patchy in terms of the range and quality of experiences offered to students. They maintain that workplace assessors either lack training for their role, or have insufficient time allowed in their other professional duties to fulfil the role properly.

The competence movement, which advocates the use of occupational standards, will have a particular impact on post-registration professional development in the workplace 'training and experience' stages. The implications are that there would be a need to build a satisfactory, assessable portfolio of evidence for a higher level NVQ as going some way, or perhaps most of the way, to meeting post-registration education and practice (PREP) requirements. This holds out the possibility of constructing a single portfolio with a dual purpose assessment which satisfies the requirements of both the professional and the vocational qualification awarding body (Storey et al. 1995a,b).

This work aims to develop a curriculum that meets vocational and academic requirements to ensure that the staff of Ashworth Hospital are competent to deliver care to meet client needs. This approach is underpinned by concerns expressed in the report of the Royal College of

Nursing Consensus Conference which points out that: 'The nature and content of programmes should reflect the interface between professional and service standards and needs. They, therefore, should include: work-place assessment, self-assessment, the development of knowledge through reflection in practice, by the accumulation in professional portfolios of evidence of their learning and development through practice as well as by academic study.' (RCN 1994)

Methodology

The approach taken has been to examine the feasibility of using an occupational standards development approach. This approach is becoming more common in the professional domain, as reported in *The Future Healthcare Workforce*:

> The professional bodies are increasingly aware of the need to deliver occupational competence. The Calman report on specialist medical training, for example, states that the completion of specialist medical training should be based on assessment of competence . . .
>
> (Conroy 1996)

The use of occupational standards is typically associated with National Vocational Qualifications, although the methodology of functional analysis and standards development is being widely used within the workplace and within professional development for a range of purposes, including defining job roles, identifying training and development needs and constructing job descriptions. In fact, the medical profession is currently using this type of methodology to develop occupational standards for senior house officers, whilst other care professionals are developing core competences for professions allied to medicine, for complementary therapies and for health promotion.

There is, however, still a lack of knowledge in the NHS on how to capitalise on the NVQ/occupational standards concept. Despite its strategic importance, it has not found its way onto the managerial agenda and there is a perception that it is a 'nursing' issue. But there are compelling reasons for the NHS to give NVQs a high priority: the occupational standards methodology provides a measure of job competence; it can also be used to facilitate the development of new roles, and to develop curricula that can prepare practitioners to undertake these roles, and contribute to the development of standards which are recognised in other European countries. Developments are also occurring within the

European Community. We therefore have to consider the European dimension in our developments.

> A major obstacle to job mobility within the European Union is still the lack of transparency of qualifications . . . . Transparency aims to give access to descriptions of qualifications from other countries that are clear enough to enable their relevance to particular jobs to be judged.
>
> (NCVQ 1995)

By developing occupational standards of competence for professionals delivering a service to people with personality disorder, the work currently underway within Ashworth Hospital Authority attempts to address the aims adopted by the Council of Ministers in 1992, in that it will be:

- enabling individuals who wish to present their occupational qualifications, education and work experience clearly and effectively to potential employers through the community
- helping employers to have easy access to clear descriptions of qualifications and relevant professional experience, in order to establish the relevance of the skills of job applicants from other member states to jobs on offer.

> (NCVQ 1995)

NVQs and their Scottish equivalents (SVQs – Scottish Vocational Qualifications) have been developed from 1986 onwards. The overall aim has been to '. . . establish a coherent national structure of vocational qualifications, framed in terms of publicly-defined standards'. The model is intended to allow comparability between a wide range of different qualifications and provide coherent and flexible routes for personal progression (Wright 1993).

The work has matched current national occupational standards with the workroles of staff and has identified gaps in the framework. Standards for practice are being developed using NVQ philosophy and methodology. NVQs and national occupational standards have been developed in a number of occupational areas, and many of these may have some relevance to the work. Examples include care, core units for professions supplementary to medicine, social work, criminal justice service, and advice, guidance and psychotherapy.

Standards development

The standards have been developed through the process of functional analysis as in Figure 5.1.

Functional analysis is the process that underpins the development of national occupational standards. It is a holistic, systems-based process used to analyse whole occupations in terms of outcomes and the purpose of work activities rather than specific activities, procedures and methods. This approach results in the development of a functional map that is presented as a 'fallen tree' as illustrated below.

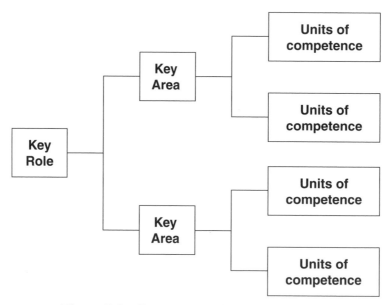

Figure 5.1   Components of a functional map.

National occupational standards (also known as units of competence) define the level of performance required for the successful achievement of work expectations. They specify best practice, and realistic future expectations, in an employment sector and are expressed in the form of elements of competence, performance criteria and range indicators. These are then used as specifications for assessment when standards are aggregated together to form qualifications.

In order to map the care for people with a personality disorder, a number of focus groups were held with staff involved in delivering or managing the care of this client group. The groups have involved representatives from nursing, psychology, social work, occupational therapy, social therapy, psychiatry and support staff.

The work to 'map the care of people with a personality disorder' originated in the Personality Disorder Unit at Ashworth Hospital, where they were attempting to identify the core competences needed by nursing staff to work with this group (Melia *et al.* 1997). Subsequently this work has been developed to include other disciplines both within Ashworth and other settings in the United Kingdom, Holland and Eire.

Focus groups have been held at Ashworth, Rampton, Broadmoor, the State Mental Hospital in Scotland, the Henderson Clinic and with colleagues at the Central Mental Hospital in Dublin and in Ministry of Justice clinics in Holland. The groups have been used to identify the key purpose of the service provided for these patients.

The draft key purpose statement which has been developed is:

> To provide safe, secure and motivating conditions in which, through the use of consistent and coherent approaches, therapeutic interventions and planned interactions, the impact of the individual's personality disorder can be minimised and they are encouraged and supported to effect a positive change in the way that they perceive, interpret and interact within their social environment.

The statement summarises the unique nature of care delivery for this patient group, and reflects the values which underpin care delivery and any inherent balances or conflicts which affect the work, such as differences between the needs of patients and the expectations of society.

The key purpose is then broken down into successive levels of detail which describe more and more precisely what it is that is expected of people. The second stage of analysis identifies key areas that are as follows:

1 promote and implement principles which underpin effective, quality practice
2 assess, develop, implement, evaluate and improve programmes of care for individuals
3 develop, implement, evaluate and improve environments and relationships which promote therapeutic goals and limit risks
4 provide and improve resources and services which facilitate organisational functioning
5 develop the knowledge, competence and practice of self and others.

Staff development

The majority of healthcare professionals who work in this specialised area of forensic mental health in the UK have had little or no specific

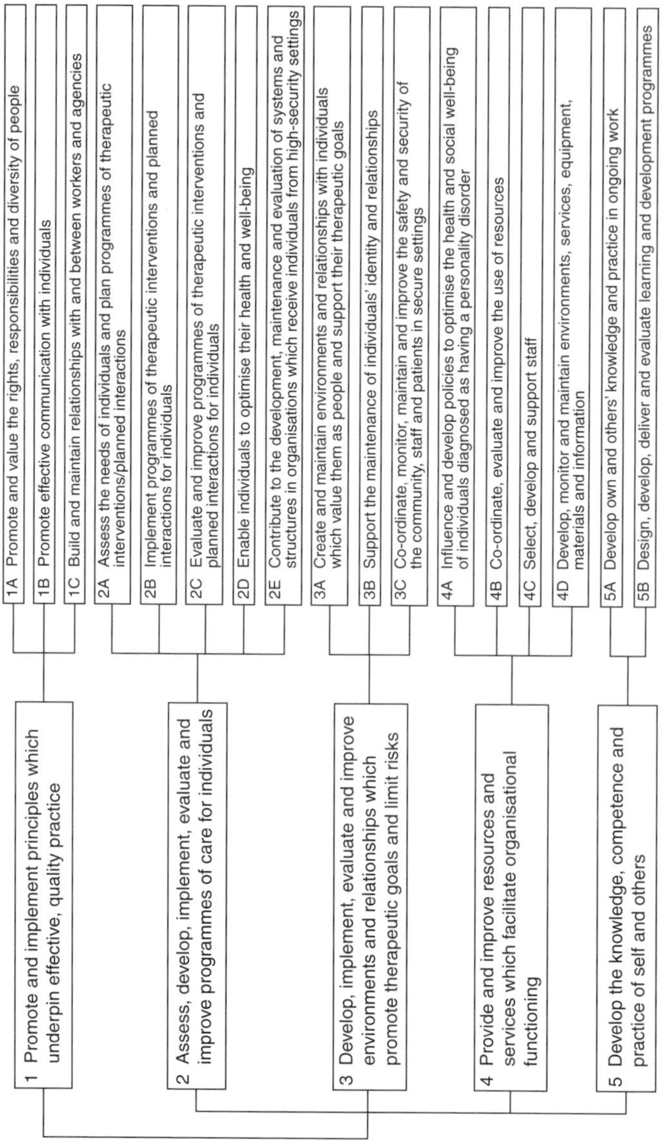

1 Promote and implement principles which underpin effective, quality practice

- 1A Promote and value the rights, responsibilities and diversity of people
- 1B Promote effective communication with individuals
- 1C Build and maintain relationships with and between workers and agencies

2 Assess, develop, implement, evaluate and improve programmes of care for individuals

- 2A Assess the needs of individuals and plan programmes of therapeutic interventions/planned interactions
- 2B Implement programmes of therapeutic interventions and planned interactions for individuals
- 2C Evaluate and improve programmes of therapeutic interventions and planned interactions for individuals
- 2D Enable individuals to optimise their health and well-being
- 2E Contribute to the development, maintenance and evaluation of systems and structures in organisations which receive individuals from high-security settings

3 Develop, implement, evaluate and improve environments and relationships which promote therapeutic goals and limit risks

- 3A Create and maintain environments and relationships with individuals which value them as people and support their therapeutic goals
- 3B Support the maintenance of individuals' identity and relationships
- 3C Co-ordinate, monitor, maintain and improve the safety and security of the community, staff and patients in secure settings

4 Provide and improve resources and services which facilitate organisational functioning

- 4A Influence and develop policies to optimise the health and social well-being of individuals diagnosed as having a personality disorder
- 4B Co-ordinate, evaluate and improve the use of resources
- 4C Select, develop and support staff
- 4D Develop, monitor and maintain environments, services, equipment, materials and information

5 Develop the knowledge, competence and practice of self and others

- 5A Develop own and others' knowledge and practice in ongoing work
- 5B Design, develop, deliver and evaluate learning and development programmes

Figure 5.2 The functional map of care for personality disorder.

preparation for working with people with a personality disorder before commencing in the job. The changes in pre-registration education, particularly nursing, make it difficult for nurses to gain experience in working with these patients. The pre-registration diploma in nursing mental health only allows 18 months in which students can develop generic mental health nursing skills. This, coupled with a dearth of clinical placements where students can work with patients with a severe personality disorder available to higher education institutions, results in difficulties for organisations managing these patients, who then have to purchase or provide additional education and training.

Most organisations, including the high-security hospitals, provide a wide range of post-registration education opportunities, either in-house or purchased from other providers. Many of these programmes have exit awards, from in-house certificates of attendance through to degrees. However, there are currently no qualifications that are based on the competences required to work with this patient group. The development of the functional map of care for people with a personality disorder has provided a basis for the development of competency-based qualifications, and assisted in the identification of a curriculum for continuing professional development of staff.

The key purpose, key roles and units of competence identified in the map have assisted in the identification of eight principal curriculum themes:

1 Boundaries and inter-relatedness
2 Management
3 Ethics
4 Communication
5 Assessment and care management
6 Research and evidence-based practice
7 Safety and security
8 Theories of personality disorder and therapeutic interventions.

These curriculum themes have been used to develop the framework of qualifications for staff at different levels and from different disciplines within the care team. Modules have been developed at Masters level to produce a postgraduate certificate. Modules are also available at a certificate in higher education level. It is anticipated that a range of academic levels will also be developed through to a Masters degree.

The use of an outcomes-based approach means that modes of delivery can be varied. Candidates will be able to use accreditation of prior learning and prior experience. The framework of qualifications will have multiple access and multiple exit points and will be awarded on the basis of assessment of portfolios that link theory to applied practice based on the occupational standards framework.

The development of a framework of occupational standards, and qualifications, has provided opportunities for the development of the staff as well as providing a vehicle for developing standards for service delivery. Candidates who have undertaken the programme have developed portfolios of evidence derived from practice. Through constructing portfolios the candidates have compared their practice with the current evidence base and examined their own approaches to service delivery and therefore have enhanced patient care.

Storey and Haigh (2002) suggest that competency-based frameworks have the potential to bring the best of both worlds together (learning theories and learning on the job), through the development of programmes of learning which:

1   assess theory through application in practice
2   subject practice to scrutiny
3   allow practitioners to reflect on appropriateness of actions taken and alternatives to be considered.

Occupational standards for assessment and therapeutic approaches to personality disorder

The following occupational standards have been incorporated within the modules that make up the postgraduate certificate and university certificate, developed by the Faculty of Health, University of Central Lancashire, which have been undertaken by nurses, psychologists, social therapists, prison officers, occupational therapists and education staff within Ashworth Hospital, medium secure units in north-west England and HMP Whitemoor in Cambridgeshire.

- **1A2: Promote people's equality, diversity and rights**
    This unit is about promoting the equality and diversity of people and their rights and responsibilities. Due to the often sensitive nature of the information about people with which the sector deals, the promotion of confidentiality is also included. The practitioner is expected to be proactive in promoting: people's rights and responsibilities; equality and diversity; people's right to confidentiality.
    Balancing individuals' rights and responsibilities with those of others (staff, other patients, visitors, etc.) is key.

- **2A2: Assess individuals to determine their overall needs and risk**

  This unit is about the initial assessment of an individual's overall needs (including health and social care and any specific therapeutic interventions that may be needed to address particular issues) and, implicitly, the risk that they pose. This may take place once the individual has been admitted (e.g. to an admission ward) or could be partly or wholly undertaken before they arrive.

  The standards need to reflect the complex nature of individuals' conditions and needs – the fact that they may be resistant to their diagnosis and to assessment (and also to their admission and/or to the notion of treatment) and that the initial period following admission may well be particularly stressful and disruptive for them.

- **2A5: Assist in the assessment of, and the planning of programmes of care for, individuals**

  This unit is about contributing to the formulation of packages of care to meet clients' assessed needs. The term 'assist in' is used to recognise that the practitioner is operating as a member of a care team, and is therefore not solely responsible for the assessment and planning process. This involves contributing to the assessment of individuals' needs, reporting and processing the outcomes of the assessment, and contributing to the planning of suitable care packages to meet the assessed needs of individuals. This is part of the care management function and is relevant for those who work with other staff to identify the complex needs of individuals or undertake simple needs-led assessments themselves.

- **2A6: Plan specific therapeutic interventions to enable individuals diagnosed as having a personality disorder to recognise and address their socially-unacceptable behaviour**

  This unit is about the planning of approaches, therapeutic activities and interactions that are specifically designed to enable the patient to recognise and address their behaviour. It is potentially a specialist unit for working with personality-disorder (PD) patients and would include extensive knowledge requirements related to the condition, its effect on individuals and the range of therapies and approaches that can be taken. It is related to unit 2A5, but that relates more to contributing to the multi-disciplinary planning of programmes of care to meet an individual's overall needs.

  The therapeutic interventions may cover a wide range of different types of therapeutic activity (psychotherapy, role playing, discussions) and may be on an individual or group basis.

- **2B3: Contribute to the joint implementation and monitoring of programmes of care for individuals**

  The term 'contribute to' is used to recognise that the practitioner is operating as a member of a care team, and is therefore not solely responsible for implementing and monitoring programmes. This unit recognises the importance of co-ordination and coherence in working with people with PD. It is designed to be applicable to all members of the multi-disciplinary team who are involved in caring for, and managing the care of, people with PD. It will include communication and sharing of information across the team and monitoring own and others' approaches to patients to ensure consistency with other team members and with the care plan. Observation, recording and reporting are important aspects of monitoring and reviewing the care programme, which will be reflected in the unit.

- **2B4: Implement specific therapeutic interventions to enable individuals to manage behaviour**

  This unit follows on from 2A6, in which therapeutic interventions are planned. Different members of the multi-disciplinary team are involved in implementing a range of different therapeutic activities and the unit needs to reflect this. Working within the limits of the individual's care programme, observing, reporting and recording will all feature.

- **2B5: Assist in the implementation and monitoring of specific therapeutic interventions**

  Similar to unit 2B4, this unit, however, reflects a lower level of responsibility and autonomy. Here, the practitioner would be assisting (e.g. through observation and recording, preparing and providing resources) rather than leading the activities and would be working under the guidance or direction of another.

- **2C2: Contribute to the evaluation and improvement of programmes of care for individuals**

  This unit is designed to be applicable to practitioners from a range of different disciplines. The term 'programme of care' has been used to mean the whole process of care designed for the individual and its evaluation, review and modification. Within the overall programme, a number of specific interventions will take place and these will also need to be planned, implemented and evaluated. The standards in this unit describe those outcomes which are common across the process. This means that the knowledge, understanding and skills which different practitioners require would depend on their own particular area of expertise and this will vary between different practitioner groups. The term 'contribute to' is used to recognise that the practitioner is operating as a member of a care team, and is therefore not solely responsible for evaluating and improving programmes.

- **2C3: Audit the quality and outcomes of others' assessment and care planning processes**

  This unit has been designed to capture the role of practitioners who review and evaluate the outcomes of another practitioner's assessment and care planning processes. This evaluation and review may be as part of an ongoing programme of peer review and quality improvement, or may be undertaken by a service manager in cases where an organisation wishes to evaluate a specific case. The person undertaking the evaluation needs to gather and analyse information on the decisions which have been made in specific cases, evaluate the courses of action taken and finalise and report on the evaluation.

- **3A6: Build and sustain relationships with individuals to reinforce their therapeutic goals**

  This unit is about establishing and maintaining relationships with patients which motivate, encourage and support them to achieve their therapeutic goals, and which model those goals. Issues of boundaries are important, as is the need for consistency, both between interactions with the patient and between members of the care team.

- **4C4: Support staff in maintaining their identity and safe personal boundaries**

  An important part of working with personality disorder is the maintenance of personal and professional identity and value by every member of the care team. There is a need to be constantly aware of manipulation, splitting, collusion, etc. and to monitor all practitioners' maintenance of identity and boundaries. This unit is not designed to be solely for management roles, as all staff have a role to play in contributing to the maintenance of coherence and consistency and reinforcing other team members' values and identities.

- **5A1: Contribute to the development of knowledge and practice**

  This unit focuses on the interaction of the practitioner with their colleagues, through exchanging information and advice, generating solutions to problems and issues in practice, and contributing to the development of others from one's own experience. 'Others' may be practitioners from the same discipline, those from other disciplines and colleagues working in the same organisation or in another. This unit is intended to be relevant to all members of multi-disciplinary teams.

- **5A2: Develop oneself within the role**

  This unit is about developing one's own knowledge and practice – a key part of the role. This involves reflecting on and evaluating one's own values, interests, priorities and effectiveness in practice, and learning from this. It is also about incorporating and embedding new knowledge into one's practice. The new knowledge may come from reflecting on and evaluating one's own practice or from finding out about and utilising the developments made by others. The unit is intended to support good practice in action research and promote effective practice. It is designed to be relevant across a multi-disciplinary team.

6

Case study 3:
Competency profiling in health informatics

Introduction

The NHS Information Authority produced a health informatics competency profile (HICP) relating to informatics skills necessary for the implementation of the *Information for Health* strategy document (DoH 1998a). This was then used in a survey designed to cover the full range of professional staff groups in the NHS and all of the topics contained in *Information for Health*.

The survey was based around two surveys, using the following staff roles:

- **General Medical Practitioner, General Dental Practitioner and Hospital Medical Staff Career Grade** (including Consultant, Associate Specialist, Staff Grade)
- **Other Doctors** (including Hospital Staff Junior Grades: Senior Registrar, Registrar, Senior House Officer, House Officer)
- **Midwifery, Health Visitor and Registered Nursing** (including Adult Nurse, Mental Health Nurse, Children's Nurse, School Nurse, Occupational Nurse, Practice Nurse)
- **Healthcare Assistant** (all student healthcare support, including unqualified/training grades)
- **Professions Allied to Medicine** (including Chiropodist, Pharmacist, Optician, Radiographer, Dietician, Podiatrist, Therapist – all disciplines, Dental Nurse and Hygienist)

- **Professional and Technical** (including Scientific and Technical staff, Paramedic, Radiologist, Patient Transport staff)
- **Executive and Senior Manager** (including Chair, Chief Executive, Medical Director, Director of Public Health, Board Member and Senior Managers who report directly to a Director)
- **Other Managers** (Departmental and Operational Managers who report to Senior Managers)
- **Senior Secretary** (Personal Assistant and Senior Secretary – non-medical)
- **Medical Secretary**
- **Other Secretary/Administration** (non-medical Junior Secretaries and Administration staff)
- **Clerical** (including Clerks and Coders – all disciplines)
- **Senior Information Manager** (Senior Managers who specialise in Information Management, including Librarians)
- **Middle Information Manager** (Other Managers who specialise in Information Management, including Librarians)
- **Information Management Specialist** (non-management staff who specialise in Information Management, including Librarians)
- **Senior Information Technology Manager** (Senior Managers who specialise in Information Technology)
- **Middle Information Technology Manager** (Other Managers who specialise in Information Technology)
- **Information Technology Specialist** (non-management staff who specialise in Information Technology)

The survey covered the full range of health informatics topics contained in HICP as follows:

- Basic Computing
- Personal Computers
  - Peripheral Equipment
  - File Management
  - Networked Facilities
- Basic Applications
- Word Processing
  - Spreadsheets
  - Databases
  - Presentations
  - Electronic Mail
  - Internet Browsing
  - Time Management
- Computer Systems
- Clinical Systems

- Non-clinical Systems
- Management Systems
- Data Quality
- Data Collection
  - Coding
  - Data Analysis
  - Data Audit
  - Data Standards
- Information Management
- Identifying Information Needs
  - Obtaining Information
  - Evaluating Information
  - Interpretation
  - Decision-making
  - Communicating Results
- System Development
- Requirements Analysis
  - Applications Development
  - Integrated Systems/Interfaces
  - Technical Standards
  - Technical Management
  - System Implementation
- Strategic Development
- Strategic Planning
  - Local Healthcare Priorities
  - Working With Partners
  - Business Cases
  - Programme/Project Management
  - Options Appraisal
  - Procurement
  - Resource Planning
  - Change Management
  - Organisational Development
  - Healthcare Process Re-design
  - Evaluation/Benefits Realisation
  - New Technology Awareness
  - e-commerce/e-business
- Clinical Informatics
- Clinical Record Keeping
  - Clinical Decision Support
  - Clinical Communications
  - Clinical Audit
  - Evidence-based Practice

- Communications Technologies
- Electronic Data Interchange
  - Links To Other Organisations
  - Voice Communications Systems
  - Network Architectures
- Security & Confidentiality
- Legislation
  - Caldicott Guardian
  - Professional Practice
  - Local Policies & Protocols
  - Security Mechanisms
  - Standards
- Knowledge Management
- Information Searches
  - Databases/Library Services
  - Patient/Public Information
  - National Infrastructure
  - Case Studies
  - Research
- Health Informatics Skills
- Reviewing HIS Skills
  - User Support
  - Health Informatics ETD.

Competency levels

The questionnaires used the competency levels contained in HICP to assess the skill and knowledge levels in health informatics for each staff group, as defined below.

Table 6.1 HICP skill levels.

Code	Level	Definition
0	None	No skills or knowledge are required in this topic
1	Basic	A basic awareness and few, if any, skills
2	Intermediate	Moderate skills and knowledge
3	Advanced	Specialist skills and knowledge
4	Expert	Full skills and knowledge

The HICP defines their competency levels as follows:

A competency level of 0 (None) indicates that a respondent has no skills or knowledge in a particular health informatics topic.

A competency level of 1 (Basic) indicates that a respondent has fundamental knowledge only, with few basic skills at most, in a particular health informatics topic. For example, the ability to switch on a personal computer and use a computer mouse to activate Basic Applications, coupled with the inability to change the displayed time or layout of the screen, would represent a basic competency in personal computers.

A competency level of 2 (Intermediate) indicates that a respondent has moderate skills and knowledge in a particular health informatics topic. For example, the ability to type a letter, insert a table, change the font size and alter the margins, coupled with an inability to alter column widths in a table or add or amend headers and footers, would represent an intermediate competency in word processing.

A competency level of 3 (Advanced) indicates that a respondent has specialist skills and knowledge in a particular health informatics topic. This means an understanding and/or ability to use a particular health informatics topic in enough detail to fully carry out a particular job role without specialist support or supervision. For example, the ability to activate electronic mail, type a message, insert an attachment, address and send the message to the intended recipients represents an advanced competency in electronic mail.

A competency level of 4 (Expert) indicates that a respondent has full skills and knowledge in a particular health informatics topic. This means a *complete* understanding and/or ability to use *all* aspects of the particular topic. In addition to the above example of advanced competency in electronic mail, respondents with expert competency would be able to add new users, allocate and change passwords, analyse and solve e-mail network problems, etc.

The expert health informatics competency level (4) applies only to information management and information technology staff (health informatics specialists), rather than clinical, managerial or administration staff. This may change as the implementation of *Information for Health* continues.

Consider as an example the competency profile for a general practitioner.

Table 6.2   GP competency profile.

Competency Area	Required Skill Level
Basic Computing	
Personal Computers	2 (Intermediate)
Peripheral Equipment	2 (Intermediate)
File Management	2 (Intermediate)
Networked Facilities	2 (Intermediate)
Basic Applications	
Word Processing	2 (Intermediate)
Spreadsheets	2 (Intermediate)
Databases	2 (Intermediate)
Presentations	2 (Intermediate)
Electronic Mail	3 (Advanced)
Internet Browsing	2 (Intermediate)
Time Management	2 (Intermediate)
Computer Systems	
Clinical Systems	2 (Intermediate)
Non-clinical Systems	1 (Basic)
Management Systems	1 (Basic)
Data Quality	
Coding	3 (Advanced)
Data Analysis	3 (Advanced)
Audit	2 (Intermediate)
Data Standards	3 (Advanced)
Information Management	
Identifying Information Needs	3 (Advanced)
Obtaining Information	3 (Advanced)
Evaluating Information	3 (Advanced)
Interpretation	3 (Advanced)
Decision-making	3 (Advanced)
Communicating Results	3 (Advanced)
System Development	
Project Management	1 (Basic)
Requirements Analysis	2 (Intermediate)
Applications Development	1 (Basic)
Integrated Systems/Interfaces	1 (Basic)
Technical Standards	1 (Basic)
System Procurement	1 (Basic)
Technical Management	1 (Basic)
System Implementation	1 (Basic)

Strategic Development

Strategic Planning	2 (Intermediate)
Local Healthcare Priorities	3 (Advanced)
Working with Partners	3 (Advanced)
Business Cases	1 (Basic)
Programme/Project Management	1 (Basic)
Options Appraisal	1 (Basic)
Strategic Procurement	1 (Basic)
Resource Planning	2 (Intermediate)
Change Management	2 (Intermediate)
Organisational Development	1 (Basic)
Healthcare Process Re-design	1 (Basic)
Evaluation / Benefits Realisation	1 (Basic)
New Technology Awareness	1 (Basic)
e-Commerce / e-Business	0

Clinical Informatics

Clinical Record Keeping	3 (Advanced)
Clinical Decision Support	3 (Advanced)
Clinical Communications	3 (Advanced)
Clinical Audit	3 (Advanced)
Evidence-based Practice	3 (Advanced)

Communications Technologies

Electronic Data Interchange	1 (Basic)
Links to Other Organisations	2 (Intermediate)
Voice Communications Systems	2 (Intermediate)
Network Architectures	3 (Advanced)

Security & Confidentiality

Legislation	3 (Advanced)
Caldicott Guardian	3 (Advanced)
Professional Practice	3 (Advanced)
Local Policies & Protocols	3 (Advanced)
Security Mechanisms	1 (Basic)
Standards	2 (Intermediate)

Knowledge Management

Information Searches	3 (Advanced)
Databases/Library Services	3 (Advanced)
Public Information	3 (Advanced)
National Infrastructure	3 (Advanced)
Case Studies	2 (Intermediate)
Research	2 (Intermediate)
Reviewing HIS Skills	1 (Basic)
User Support	1 (Basic)
Health Informatics ETD	2 (Intermediate)

The *National Health Informatics Competency Annual Survey* was carried out by the National Health Service Information Authority (NHSIA) in line with NHS Executive policy, based on recommendations from the National Audit Office. Further annual surveys are planned until 2005.

The report concludes that there is an:

> . . . enormous challenge facing the Health Service if it is to meet the targets of and successfully implement *Information for Health* in the stated time frame (i.e. by 2005).
>
> Whilst the results indicate that there are 'pockets of excellence' around the country, they are few and far between. For example, most management, secretarial and HIS staff have the required levels of competency in personal computers and knowledge of security mechanisms but with the exception of senior IT staff, little in information management.
>
> A glance at appendices J and K (which summarise the overall results in terms of the gaps that exist between the target levels and current levels of competencies) shows just how big the challenge is.
>
> With few exceptions, the majority of NHS professional staff requires some level of education, training and development (ETD) in almost all health informatics topics. For example:
>
> Most medical staff do not meet the recommended levels of competency in any of the topics, with the sole exception of GMP/GDP/Hospital Medical Staff Career Grade, who have the required basic knowledge of security mechanisms.
>
> Most other clinical staff, which includes the largest numbers (of around ½ million staff), do not meet the recommended levels of competency in any of the topics.

The full reports, both profile and survey, are available (at the time of writing) online from the NHSIA's website at http://www.nhsia.nhs.uk.

Conclusions

This profile and survey represents a major exercise in competency profiling. It has highlighted a major training need in relation to informatics skills. However, there are a number of problems with the methodology adopted.

- The roles used fail to take proper account of the specialist information needs of clinicians, especially specific groups, e.g. NHSDirect nurses.
- The levels of competency appeared to be defined in an *ad hoc* way.
- The use of self-assessment in the survey raises questions about the reliability of the data. However, it seems likely that self-assessment will provide an over-optimistic set of results, and in light of the conclusions about the training needs, this seems unlikely to have an effect on the conclusions.

As the Authority is committed to making an annual survey until 2005, this provides the opportunity to develop and improve the methodology. In the following chapters, we shall develop an alternative strategy to look at the implementation of electronic health records and the consequent training needs.

Applying the HICP in a local context

In order to really understand the processes involved in assessing an individual's competency profile using this model, perhaps it is easiest to 'walk through' the various processes. For this exercise we will use some of the NHSIA competencies that have already been developed relating to informatics and the skills required by staff if *Information for Health* is to be fully implemented.

As outlined previously, it is probably easiest to imagine the competency model as a grid, either a draughtboard or a spreadsheet depending upon your level of expertise, into which we can slot three types of information.

1   The roles which people perform (the side of the board/rows on the spreadsheet).
2   The area of skills or knowledge or behaviour required (the top of the board or the columns on the spreadsheet).
3   The level which is required for each combination of the above (the squares of the board or the cells on the spreadsheet).

So, we need to actually put some information into the framework so that a comparison can be made between an individual's level of performance and that which is expected or required from someone undertaking that role within their organisation.

The first thing that needs to be fitted onto our framework is a list of all of the possible roles which each individual may play. This is a key stage in the process as the degree of specification applied now fundamentally affects the whole process. The key is to ensure that each individual role is clearly specified so that it can be related directly to an individual's job or role within the organisation. The greater the number of different and specific roles which are added, the more exact the match to the individual's role. Against this must be set the time and complexity of data design and entry which comes from an increase in the number of roles.

If we look at primary care as an example this may become a little clearer. A simple way to determine which roles we are going to specify would be to directly link our role definitions to job titles. Thus we could add in to our model the following roles:

- General Practitioner
- Practice Manager
- Practice Receptionist
- Practice Nurse
- Health Visitor
- Community Midwife
- District Nurse
- etc.

These would each then have their own row of squares in the model. There are problems with specifying roles as broad as this, but not as many as classifying all qualified nurses, midwifes and health visitors as a single group, or all allied health professionals to another, as happens in the NHSIA competency framework outlined below. This is not to say that the idea of grouping several roles into one for a particular competency area is wrong. Rather, that the model is designed to be used for the full range of clinical, professional and administrative aspects of each individual role. If this is the case, then each role must clearly be allocated its own row of squares or cells in the model. Without this specificity there is no accurate benchmark against which each individual can be assessed. If the model was to be used in isolation to look solely at one area of competency then it may well be sufficient to group a number of roles together when they have shared skills requirements. Such use, though, would be to ignore the full benefits available from the model.

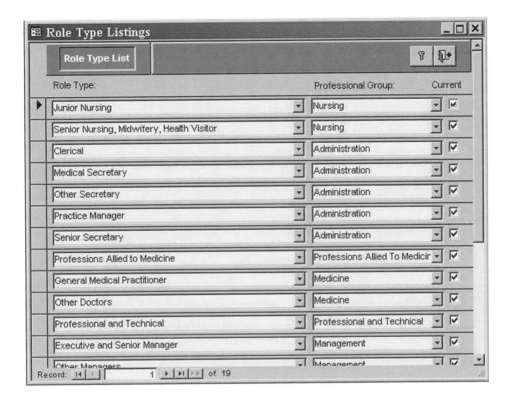

Now we have a list of roles that, in the model, act as labels or names for a row of squares or cells. This is our queue of people lined up at the side of the draughtboard. You will see that we have also added to each role a description of which professional group they belong to. This enables the system to analyse needs not only at the individual and role level but also at the professional level. We have also included whether or not that role is currently in use. This allows the system to force new staff to be allocated only a current role and not an historical one such as leech keeper.

The next stage is to define the columns of squares or cells across the top of our board/spreadsheet.

The key stage here is to specify what are the skills, knowledge or behaviour against which you wish to measure each individual's perform-ance. Not the level of performance that is required, but the actual skill to be measured. Each of these items will act as the label to a column of squares or cells. You will see from the screen below that we also include some additional information about each item.

To facilitate the assessment process, each competency item is given a simple descriptive name and a much more detailed description. Each item is also given an index number, to allow for easy identification, and a competency area.

By grouping together a number of similar competency items into a competency area it is possible to analyse the data collected at a higher level. So rather than just looking at performance in word processing, we can examine a number of items such as word processing, spreadsheets, databases, etc. all together as 'Basic Applications'.

The first stage in this part of the process is to identify the general or broad types of competency that we are interested in and, most importantly, the rating scale that we intend to use to measure the degree of skill with which each competency is performed. You will see from the screen below that in the case of the *Information for Health* competencies we are using the NHSIA rating scale.

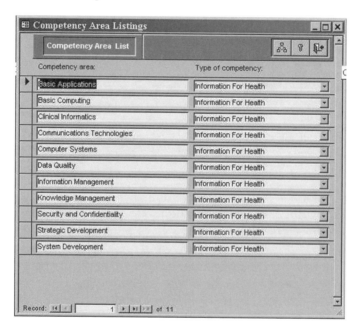

Next we must divide each of these general types into more specific areas of competency. Remember, we are not writing the competencies as behavioural statements, 'can do x, y or z', but as an item in which the individual is expected to perform.

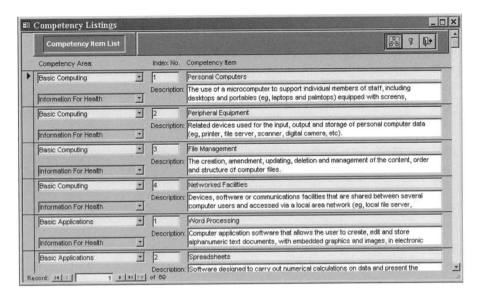

We are now nearing the final stage of setting up the system. So far we have added roles to one side of the model and competency items to the other. The last task is to fill in the intersecting squares. These then become the benchmarks for the level of performance that is required by each sort of person in each competency area. This is setting the markers on our test-your-strength machines in each square of our draughtboard. In addition, we have allocated a 'criticality' level to each competency. This allows the training needs, once they are identified, to be ranked in importance rather than just alphabetically.

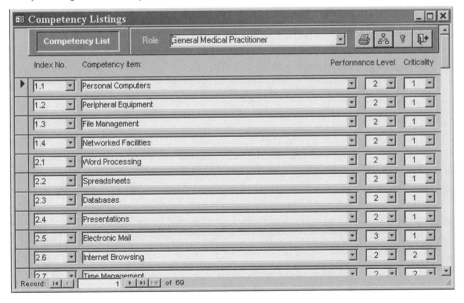

Now, imagine yourself to be a general practitioner in an inner city practice. You log onto the system and search for your record. Obviously, you will only be allowed to see the records you are entitled to, i.e. your own!

Having selected your record, you check that your details are still correct. The vital pieces of information, other than your name of course, are your workplace and your professional role . . .

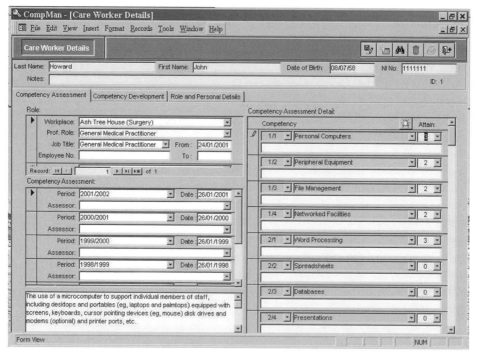

. . . you then enter the details required for this assessment – essentially, who is assessing your competency, which may be just you if this is going to be a self-assessment, and today's date. The system will then do the clever bit of selecting the appropriate row of competency items for your role before displaying these as a list down the right hand side of the screen. Hidden in the background are the benchmarks for each of these competencies that make up your job.

For each of the competency items, together with your assessor if you have one, you come to a decision as to your performance level against that individual item and score it either as the numerical value or by selecting the textual description. In order to help you make up your mind there are a couple of aids. For instance, the descriptions of what is meant by each level are available as a separate help screen and in the bottom left of the screen is a more detailed description of what is meant by the competency title.

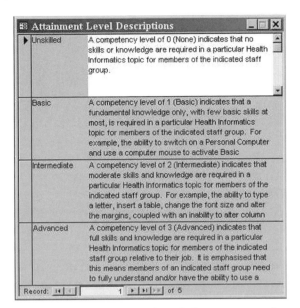

In the underlying database there is the ability to record not one but two values for this performance level for situations where the users wish to have this option available. Usually the availability of the 'Comments' box is enough to deal with disagreements between assessed and assessor.

Having selected the appropriate performance level from the scale, the process is then repeated for each of the competencies to be assessed. Once all of these are completed, the individual has a measure of their performance, both in absolute terms of the skill measure used and relative to the levels that are required for each aspect of their role.

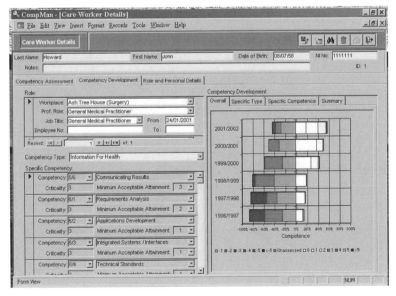

This analysis of training needs is presented in a number of ways, firstly as a graph (see previous page). Each bar represents all of the competencies assessed on a particular date. The X-axis is scaled so that 0 is in the mid-point. The proportion of the bar to the right or left of the 0 indicates the proportion of competencies above or below the level required by somebody working in that role. The colour coding of the bar represents the actual amount by which this minimum acceptable level is under- or overachieved. Each assessment of competency is shown as an individual bar on the graph, with the most recent at the top. By showing this as a series of bars it is clear at a glance how the individual's overall level of competence is progressing over time.

Secondly, performance can be shown against an individual competence over time (see below). Here the X-axis is again set with 0 as the mid-point. A score of 0 indicates that the individual is at the level required in their role for the selected competence. Values to the right indicate 'over' performance whilst values to the left of 0 indicate 'under' performance and thus development need.

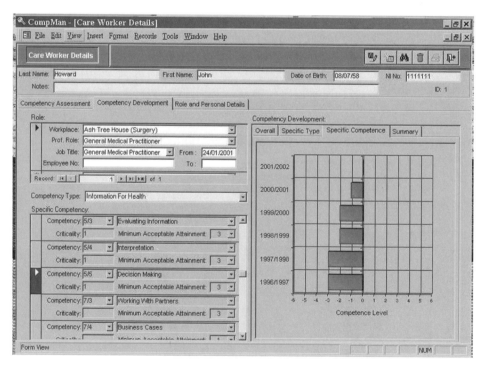

These graphs look very pretty (if you like that sort of thing!) and are helpful in giving an impression of how well you are performing against your benchmark. However, for a more detailed report on your performance, a text list of performance scores against the minimum required competence is available for this or any other selected appraisal (see below).

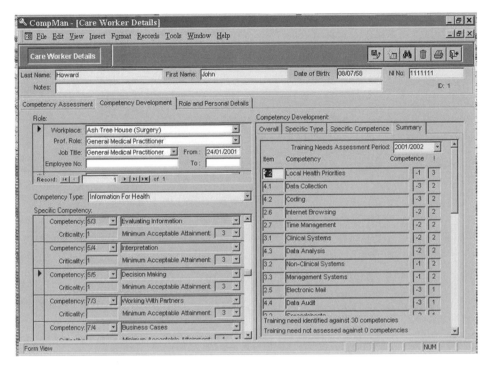

This is also available as a printed report that shows the gap between their actual and required performance and outlines possible ways in which the needs identified may be met.

For managers and human resources staff, the data from your appraisal and that of your colleagues is available to show exactly who needs what training. Obviously, access to your details is controlled so that only those people who need to know your details are allowed to do so. However, anonymous data of the training needs is then available to inform strategic as well as training decisions, both for the practice and for the wider organisation, in this case a primary care trust (see following page).

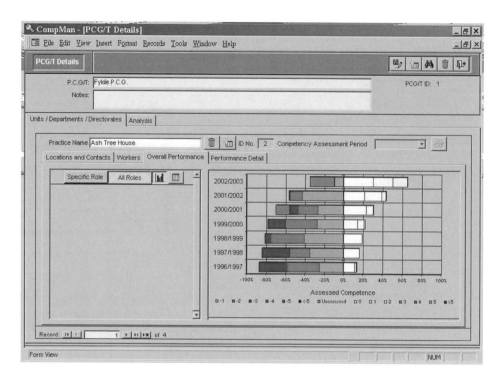

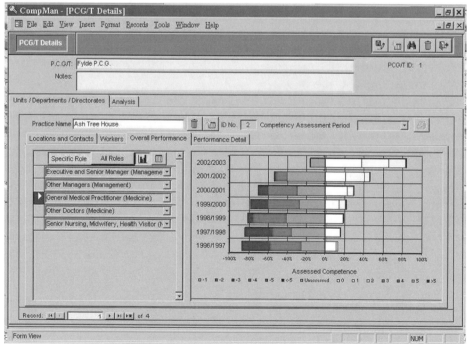

7

Linking competency to organisational development

Maturity models

Maturity models have been developed largely for quality assurance within the engineering field. However, they have been employed in a variety of applications by the authors to help with managing change. They have also been combined with training needs analysis models to enhance the power of such methods.

The first and most famous maturity model was the Process Maturity Model (PMM), which evolved into the Capability Maturity Model (CMM). This model was commissioned from the Software Engineering Institute (SEI) from Carnegie Mellon University by the US military.

The Capability Maturity Model

The basic premise underlying the SEI's maturity model is that the quality of a software product is largely determined by the quality of the software development and maintenance processes used to build it. The SEI maturity model is defined as a five-level framework for how an organisation matures its software processes from *ad hoc*, chaotic processes to mature, disciplined software processes.

Gilchrist (1992) describes the levels as shown in Table 7.1.

Table 7.1 Five levels of the SEI CMM (after Gilchrist 1992).

Level	Designation	Description
1	Initial	The organisation has undefined processes and controls.
2	Repeatable	The organisation has standardised methods facilitating repeatable processes.
3	Defined	The organisation monitors and improves its processes.
4	Managed	The organisation possesses advanced controls, metrics and feedback.
5	Optimising	The organisation uses metrics for optimisation purposes.

The model is questionnaire-based. Questions are divided into 'essentials' and 'highly desirable'. To achieve a given level, an organisation must attain 90% 'yes' answers to essential questions and 80% 'yes' answers to highly desirable questions.

The model is shown schematically in Figure 7.1:

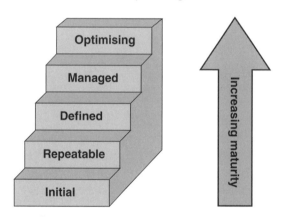

Figure 7.1 Schematic view of the Capability Maturity Model.

The software process is defined as a set of activities, methods, practices and transformations that people use to develop and maintain software and the associated products. The model assumes that as an organisation matures, the software process becomes better defined and more consistently implemented throughout the organisation. This view makes the basic principles of the maturity model approach adaptable to any management of change process.

The maturity model seeks to measure how well these processes are carried out. It may be traced directly to the work of Crosby (1979). He describes a quality management maturity grid (ibid., Chapter 3), which applies five stages to six measurement categories in subjectively rating an organisation's quality operation. The five stages are:

1 uncertainty, where management is confused and uncommitted regarding quality as a management tool
2 awakening, where management is beginning to recognise that quality management can help
3 enlightenment, when the decision is made to really conduct a formal quality improvement programme
4 wisdom, where the company has the chance to make changes permanent (things are basically quiet and people wonder why they used to have problems)
5 certainty, where quality management is considered an absolutely vital part of company management.

The six measurement categories are:

1 management understanding and attitude, characterised as 'no comprehension of quality as a management tool' at uncertainty and 'an essential part of the company system' at certainty
2 quality organisation status, characterised as hidden at uncertainty and a thought leader/main concern at certainty
3 problem handling; problems are fought when they occur at uncertainty and prevented at certainty
4 cost of quality as a percentage of sales, characterised as 20% at uncertainty and 2.5% at certainty
5 quality improvement actions, characterised as no organised activities at uncertainty and as a normal and continued activity at certainty
6 summation of company quality posture, summarised as 'we do not know why we have problems with quality' at uncertainty and 'we know why we do not have problems with quality' at certainty.

Crosby's maturity matrix is summarised in Table 7.2:

Table 7.2 Quality maturity matrix (after Crosby 1979).

	Attitude	Quality status	Problem handling	Cost as % of sales	QI actions	Posture
Uncertainty						
Awakening						
Enlightenment						
Wisdom						
Certainty						

In a precursor to the maturity model itself, Radice (1985), working with Humphrey, identified 12 process stages, which were characterised by 11 attributes measured on a five-point scale. The process stages were stages in the life cycle: requirements; product level design; component level design; module level design; code; unit test; functional verification test; product verification test; system verification test; package and release; early support programme; and general availability. The 11 attributes were: process; methods; adherence to practices; tools; change control; data gathering; data communication and use; goal setting; quality focus; customer focus; and technical awareness. The five-point scale consisted of traditional, awareness, knowledge, skill and wisdom, and integrated management system.

Humphrey brought these concepts to the Software Engineering Institute in 1986, revised them to define maturity levels, and developed the foundation for current use throughout the software industry.

The origins of the maturity model itself lie in a request to provide the Federal government with a method for assessing the capability of their software contractors.

In August 1986, the SEI, with assistance from the MITRE Corporation, began developing a process maturity framework that would assist organisations in improving their software process. In June 1987, the SEI released a brief description of the software process maturity framework (Humphrey 1987), and, in September 1987, a preliminary maturity questionnaire (Humphrey and Sweet 1987).

The 1987 SEI technical report *Characterising the Software Process: a maturity framework* (Humphrey 1987) described the software process maturity framework of the five levels in terms of the key actions needed to advance from one level to the next. These key actions were the first high-level expressions of what has become the key process areas in the CMM.

These actions are summarised in Tables 7.3 to 7.6, based upon the analysis of Paulk (1995). The model evolved through 1988 and 1989, particularly through the publication of *Managing the Software Process* (Humphrey 1989), which documented a new version of the framework.

Since then, the model has continued to evolve, as shown in Table 7.7.

Individual levels of the CMM

At level 2 of the model, an organisation is expected to have standardised methods enabling repeatable processes.

The questionnaire asks whether:

- software tools are used to support documentation
- projects are tracked
- costing and sizing are performed
- change control is implemented
- standards are used
- reviews are taking place.

Table 7.3 Key actions for moving from maturity level 1 to level 2.

Area	Required action
Project management	The fundamental role of a project management system is to ensure effective control of commitments. For software, this starts with an understanding of the magnitude of the job to be done. In the absence of such an orderly plan, no commitment can be better than an educated guess.
Management oversight	A suitably disciplined software development organisation must have corporate oversight. The lack of management reviews typically results in uneven and generally inadequate implementation of the process, as well as frequent over-commitments and cost surprises.
Product assurance	A product assurance group is charged with assuring management that the software development work is actually done the way it is supposed to be done. To be effective, the assurance organisation must have an independent reporting line to senior management and sufficient resources.
Change control	Control of changes in software development is fundamental to business and financial control as well as to technical stability. To develop quality software on a predictable schedule, the requirements must be established and maintained with reasonable stability throughout the development cycle.

Sources: (Humphrey 1987; Paulk 1995)

Table 7.4 Key actions for moving from maturity level 2 to level 3.

Area	Required action
Process group	Establish a process group. This is a technical group with exclusive focus on improving the software development process. Until someone is given a full-time assignment to work on the process, little orderly progress can be made in improving it.
Process architecture	Establish a software development process architecture, which describes the technical and management activities required for proper execution of the development process. The architecture is a structural decomposition into tasks, which each have entry criteria, functional descriptions, verification procedures and exit criteria.
Software engineering methods	If they are not already in place, introduce a family of software engineering methods and technologies. These include design and code inspections, formal design methods, library control systems and comprehensive testing methods.

Sources: (Humphrey 1987; Paulk 1995)

Table 7.5 Key actions for moving from maturity level 3 to level 4.

Area	Required action
Process measurement	Establish a minimum basic set of process measurements to identify the quality and cost parameters of each step.
Process database	Establish a process database with resources to manage and maintain it.
Process analysis	Provide sufficient process resources to analyse this data and advise project members on the data's meaning and use.
Product quality	Assess the relative quality of each product and inform management where quality targets are not being met.

Sources: (Humphrey 1987; Paulk 1995)

Table 7.6   Key actions for moving from maturity level 4 to level 5.

Area	Required action
Automated support	Provide automatic support for gathering process data.
Process optimisation	Turn the management focus from the product to the process.

Sources: (Humphrey 1987; Paulk 1995)

Table 7.7   Evolution of the CMM.

Year	Version published
1987	Software process maturity framework (Humphrey)
1987	Preliminary maturity questionnaire (Humphrey and Sweet)
1987	*Characterising the Software Process: a maturity framework* (Humphrey)
1989	*Managing the Software Process* (Humphrey)
1990	Draft version of CMM (v0.2)
1991	Version for discussion (v0.6)
1991	v1.0: *Capability Maturity Model for Software* (Paulk *et al.* 1991)
	Key Practices of the Capability Maturity Model (Weber *et al.*)
1993	v1.1: *Capability Maturity Model for Software, version 1.1* (Paulk *et al.* 1993a)
	Key Practices of the Capability Maturity Model, version 1.1 (Paulk *et al.* 1993b)

By level 3, the organisation is expected to be monitoring and improving. The questionnaire asks about:

- lessons learnt and transferred to new projects
- training programmes
- control of interfaces
- monitoring of subcontractors
- evaluation of new techniques.

At level 4, the questionnaire requires the organisation to:

- operate a database for metrics data
- set measurable quality goals
- run a tool environment
- use a model for handling defects.

At level 5, the questionnaire asks the organisation about optimisation, specifically whether:

- productivity is measured
- systems and components are re-used
- old technology is replaced
- the software process is being improved
- errors are actively prevented.

The requirements of the latest version of the CMM (v1.1) for each level are summarised in Table 7.8.

Table 7.8 Overview of requirements of CMM v1.1 (after Paulk 1995).

Maturity level			
2	*3*	*4*	*5*
Requirements Management	Organisation Process Focus	Quantitative Process Management	Defect Prevention
Software Project Planning	Organisation Process Definition	Software Quality Management	Technology Change Management
Software Tracking and Oversight	Training Programme		Process Change Management
Software Subcontract Management	Integrated Software Management		
Software Quality Assurance	Software Product Engineering		
Software Configuration Management	Intergroup Co-ordination		
	Peer Reviews		

Linking training needs to organisational development

As organisations mature, so the training needs of the staff of that organisation change. Generally, more advanced organisations require more skills from their staff. For example, we consider the following maturity model developed to monitor and improve the use of evidence in clinical practice.

Table 7.9 The Research and Development Maturity Model.

Level	Name	Description
1	*Ad hoc*	Little use of evidence
		No systematic use
2	Local guidelines	Guidelines developed in-house
		Agreed standards for use
3	External	National standards adopted
		Systematic usage and policy
4	Embedded	Monitoring of policy and usage
		Routine clinical audit and usage
		Secondary research to compile own EB guidelines
5	Originating	Commissioning or practice of primary research arising from systematic needs assessment

Then we see that skill levels required change as the organisation develops: to achieve level 2, staff need the ability to define and use guidelines, dependent upon role. By level 4, staff need the ability to assess other people's research. By level 5, they need the ability to carry out and commission their own research.

From a competency perspective this provides a training needs analysis method that reflects not only the role of the staff but the state of development of their organisation. It facilitates the prioritisation of training needs identified and ensures maximum relevance of the training needs to the individuals.

To consider this further, consider the case study in the next chapter.

8

Case study 4:
Electronic health records in primary care

The context

The role and importance of information within the NHS and particularly in primary care has grown significantly since *The New NHS* White Paper (DoH 1997) and the subsequent *Information for Health* (DoH 1998a) and *The NHS Plan: building the information core* (DoH 2000c) documents.

However, there remain a number of significant problems.

- Much of the investment has gone into hardware and high visibility projects such as the NHSNet.
- Competency levels in informatics remain low (NHSIA 2001).
- The informatics skills of clinicians have been neglected compared to those of IM&T specialists.
- Previous neglect of information management issues within the clinical context have led to data quality problems and ill-defined processes.

The GPIMM/TNAMM model was developed to provide a means for primary care to improve their skills and processes in the area of managing their clinical information to both improve patient care and meet government targets of paperless operation by 2005.

The model

The model is based around five primary maturity levels, with an additional zero as the level for non-computerised practices.

Table 8.1 Levels of the GPIMM.

Level	Designation	Summary description
0	Paper-based	The practice has no computer system.
1	Computerised	The practice has a computer system. It is used only by the practice staff.
2	Computerised PHC team	The practice has a computer system. It is used by the practice staff and the PHC team, including the doctors.
3	Coded	The system makes limited use of Read Codes.
4	Bespoke	The system is tailored to the needs of the practice through agreed coding policies and the use of clinical protocols.
5	Paperless	The practice is completely paperless, except where paper records are a legal requirement.

The maturity levels are summarised in Table 8.1.

Many practices becoming part of primary care trusts in 2001 and 2002 were still at or below level 2, even after up to ten years of computing experience. This provides a significant barrier to clinical practice developments.

The GPIMM framework provides a means for helping practices develop further to improve their usage of their systems. It should be noted that development will not, in many cases, require investment in new systems, but in extracting greater benefit from existing systems.

The overall structure of the model is shown in Figure 8.1.

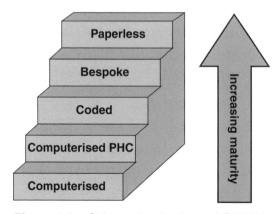

Figure 8.1 Schematic structure of GPIMM.

The activities expected at each level are shown in Table 8.2, the activity matrix.

Table 8.2 The GPIMM model matrix.

Maturity level criteria	0 Paper-based	1 Comput-erised	2 Computerised PHC team	3 Coded	4 Bespoke	5 Paper-less
Computer system installed	✗	✓	✓	✓	✓	✓
Used by practice	✗	✓	✓	✓	✓	✓
Used by doctors during consultation	✗	✗	✓	✓	✓	✓
Read Codes used	✗	✗	✗	✓	✓	✓
Standard codes used	✗	✗	✗	✗	✓	✓
Validation of codes	✗	✗	✗	✗	✓	✓
Liaison with other stakeholders	✗	✗	✗	✗	✗	✓
100% coding	✗	✗	✗	✗	✗	✓
System used to proactively manage repeat prescribing	✗	✗	✗	✓	✓	✓
System used to proactively manage acute prescribing	✗	✗	✗	✗	✓	✓
System used to proactively manage health promotion	✗	✗	✗	✗	✓	✓
System used to implement clinical protocols	✗	✗	✗	✗	✓	✓
System used to carry out real-time audits	✗	✗	✗	✗	✓	✓
IOS electronic links	✗	✗	✗	✓	✓	✓
Full use of electronic links	✗	✗	✗	✗	✗	✓
Paper records only used when legally required	✗	✗	✗	✗	✗	✓

Analysis is based around a relatively simple questionnaire. This is possible because the model has at its heart a logical model of practice information development. Practices that show different levels of maturity in different areas should consider whether those developments have occurred in a logical fashion. The presence of 'outliers', i.e. higher or lower maturity levels in one area, may be indicative of wasted efforts.

The questionnaire considers five areas to assess maturity:

- **Computerisation:** This is simply a filter to identify those practices that remain paper-based.
- **Personnel usage:** This section looks at the impact of the system upon the practice. Systems used only by practice staff are severely limited in their usefulness.
- **Coding:** This section is crucial. It considers not just the extent of coding, but the quality of coding through the extent of policies and consultation underpinning coding practice.

- **System usage:** This section is concerned with the impact that the system has upon the working methods of the practice. It measures the extent to which the system works for the practice and not the other way around.
- **Electronic patient records:** This section is concerned with the implementation of the electronic patient record. It considers how far the electronic patient record is realised both inside and outside the practice.

The philosophy within the GPIMM concerning practice development is that the raising of the maturity level of information procedure and systems is not an end in itself, but rather a means to facilitating practice development. In practice, increasing the maturity level within the GPIMM removes barriers to better clinical practice.

In particular, progress to level 3 provides many opportunities for clinical practice development with the provision of a Read Coded information resource. Further development to level 4 has a direct facilitating effect on working practices.

In Table 8.3, the key tasks required to move from one level of the GPIMM to the next are identified.

In order to support the practice development, competency sets based upon Benner's (1984) model have been defined for each GPIMM level, and for four key roles:

- doctor
- nurse
- practice manager
- administrator.

As the practice develops, so the competency level rises. For example, if a practice wishes to move to level 3 processes, so the clinicians are required to become competent in the use of Read Codes, which is not a requirement at level 2.

Level	Role	Competency					
		A	B	C	D	E	F
Level 5	Practice Manager	5	4	4	3	4	4
Level 4	Practice Manager	4	3	4	3	3	4
Level 3	Practice Manager	4	2	3	3	2	3
Level 2	Practice Manager	3	1	3	2	1	2
Level 1	Practice Manager	3	0	2	2	0	1
Level 0	Practice Manager	2	0	1	1	0	0

Figure 8.2 Varying competency requirements for increasing GPIMM levels.

Figure 8.2 shows a slice through the model, identifying the different performance levels required by a practice manager in a variety of competency items at increasing levels of GPIMM maturity. Each role has a vertical cross-section of the model. If we sliced the model horizontally through a single GPIMM level we could see, for that maturity level, the performance levels required by each role in a variety of competency areas.

Table 8.3 Key tasks to move from one GPIMM level to another.

From level	To level	Key tasks
0	1	• Procure computerised patient records system • Train practice staff • Establish age/sex register
1	2	• Persuade doctors and other PHC workers to use system in consultations • Train PHC team in use of system • Establish new working practices based around use of the system
2	3	• Persuade all staff to use Read Codes • Train all staff in use of Read Codes • Discuss scope and nature of coding
3	4	• Implement coding standards with training • Implement practice-defined protocols for diagnosis and prescribing with training • Implement computer-based health promotion policy with training • Implement real-time audits with training
4	5	• Move all records to electronic form • Agree coding standards with external bodies • Agree technology standards with other bodies

In order to provide useful tools for trusts and practices, based upon these models, the models have been incorporated into management systems for primary care trusts that facilitate both the management of change and the monitoring of staff competency.

The tools

The tools are provided as a database application, aimed at primary care trusts. The database is written in two halves. The front end is written in Access, the back end may be supplied as an Access database or in SQL Server. The back end holds all the information on practices and their staff, and the front end allow the user to access information on organisation maturity and competency. The system will hold basic data in common on staff and practices, so any number of process maturity and/or training needs models may be added, not just for information maturity but also for other areas, e.g. clinical competencies or management maturity models.

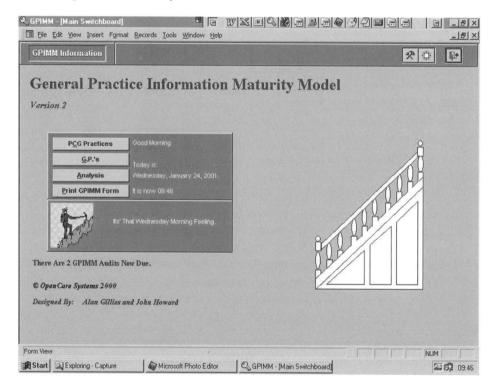

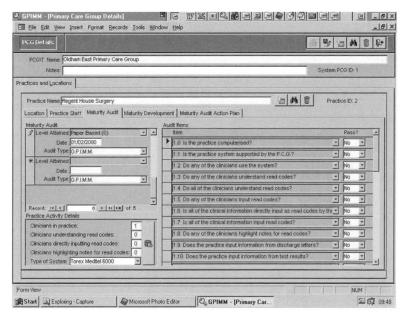

The first step in using the GPIMM/TNAMM tools after entering basic data on staff and practices is to audit the practice for information maturity. The system provides a computerised version of the GPIMM questionnaire (see above).

The computerised tool will not only provide a calculated current GPIMM level, but will identify key actions in order to achieve the next GPIMM level, and higher GPIMM levels in subsequent years.

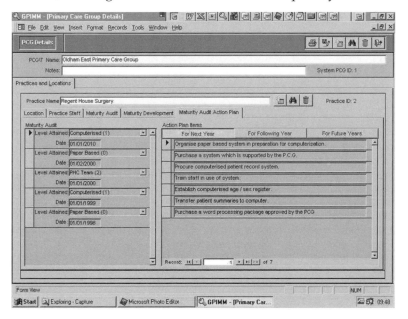

The system also provides profile information for the PCT, either for all practices or longitudinally for an individual practice.

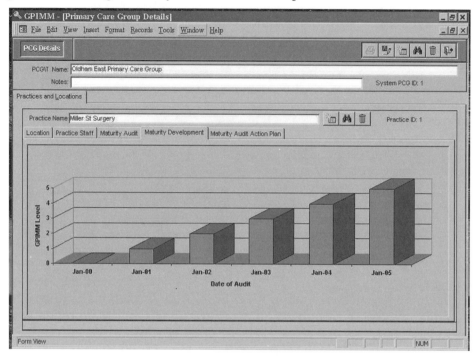

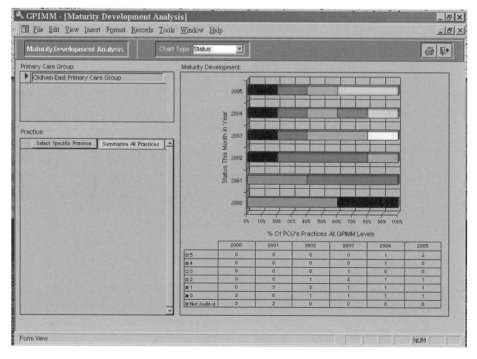

Once the practice maturity is established, this defines the competency requirements for the staff. Their current skill levels are first established through a computerised training audit. This may be done as part of an appraisal or as a self-assessment.

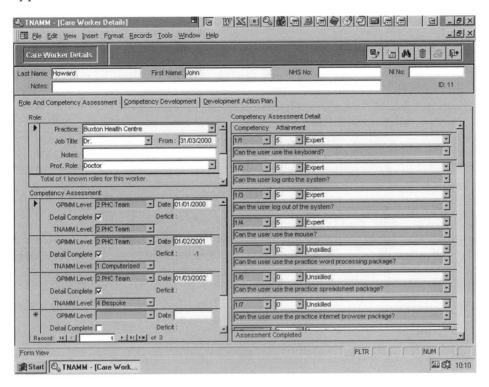

From this, their training needs may be defined as the gap between their current skills and those of a practitioner fulfilling their role in an organisation at the stage of development that their organisation has currently reached. The system defines the competency level relative to their current organisational maturity level and that required by the organisation's next target.

In addition, the tools provide summaries for management to identify the organisation's training priorities.

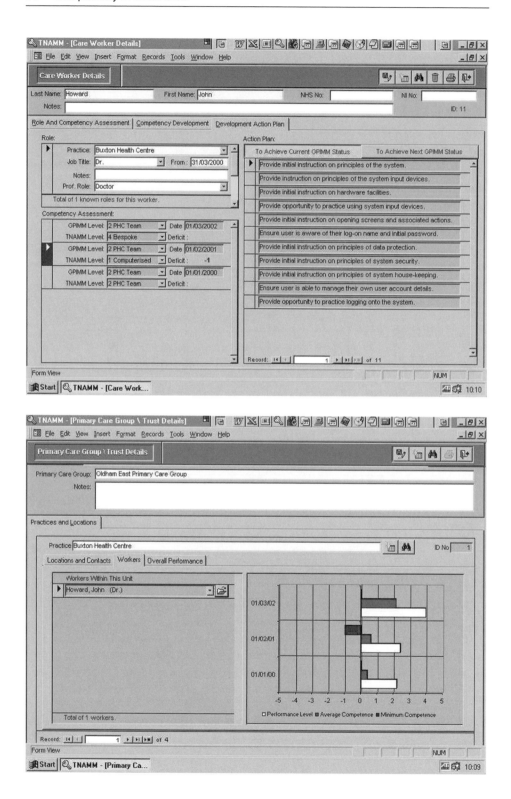

Benefits for other applications

The GPIMM/TNAMM work provides two key innovations that could usefully be applied to other domains:

- The use of maturity models to provide competency sets which are sensitive to organisational development, allowing prioritisation of training and increasing relevance for both organisations and individuals.
- The development of management tools for healthcare trusts which simplify the application of these techniques and maximise the benefits.

Work is currently underway to apply these benefits in other domains. Discussions are also currently underway with the NHSIA to inform future implementations of the annual national HICP.

More information is available online at http://www.alangillies.com.

9

Linking competency to e-learning

The future

The software tools developed for GPIMM/TNAMM provide a shell into which any process maturity and training needs model can be slotted.

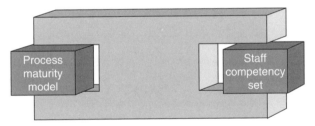

Figure 9.1 Software tools act as a shell into which different models can be slotted.

This can then be expanded further. The use of the process maturity model allows an organisation to define key milestones from its organisation strategy. These can then become the key stages of maturity development. In this way, training activity can be related directly to meeting organisational strategic goals.

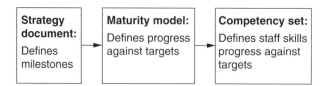

Figure 9.2 From organisational strategy to training needs.

The use of technology allows this to be taken one step further, with the training needs being linked to specific learning materials. Initially, these may be in terms of a variety of forms:

• books
• courses
• interactive e-learning materials.

However, the potential for a linked e-learning environment is seductive.

How it might work

If we take our domain as information management, then the technology already exists to define just such an integrated environment.

Let us suppose that I am a GP working in a practice. The first step would be to carry out a GPIMM audit.

The results show that the practice is currently operating at level 2.

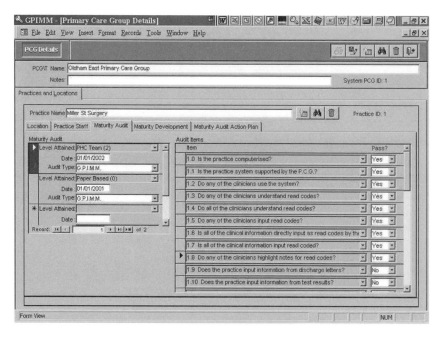

The TNAMM audit reveals that my current skill level with respect to using Read Codes to code clinical data is Advanced Beginner, which is adequate for GPIMM level 2, giving me a competence of 0, meaning that I am at the level required, given the current maturity of the practice.

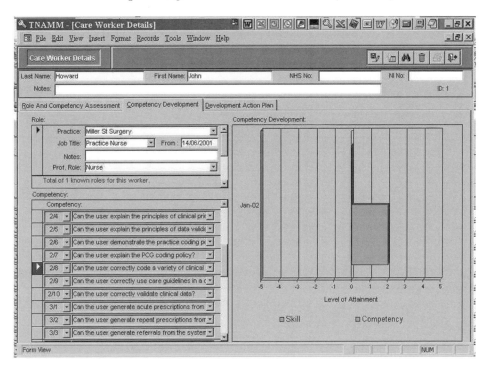

However, by next year, the practice has moved on and is now at GPIMM level 3, which requires GPs to be competent in respect of Read Codes, so even though I am just as skilful as I was last year, this is now no longer adequate, leaving me with a competency level of –1 and a respective training need.

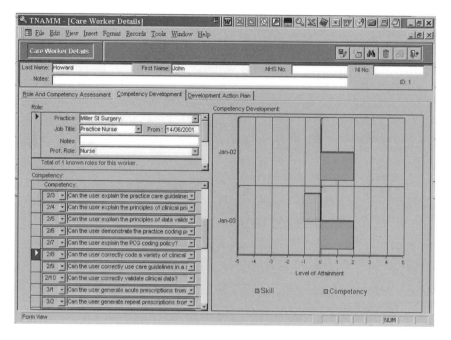

Currently the TNAMM simply defines this as a training need and offers suggestions as to the learning activities that would be appropriate to allow me to bring myself up to the increased skill level now required. This is provided as an action plan for the coming year.

However, it would be simple, in addition, to link this to a dedicated e-learning module to provide the required theoretical knowledge of Read Codes and exercises to practise the skill. This could be either a module, a reference to a book, or an on-line resource – or a dedicated e-learning module on a CD.

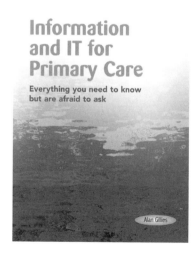

Information and IT for Primary Care

Everything you need to know but are afraid to ask

Alan Gillies

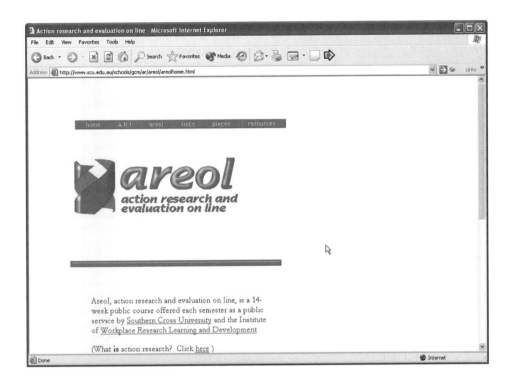

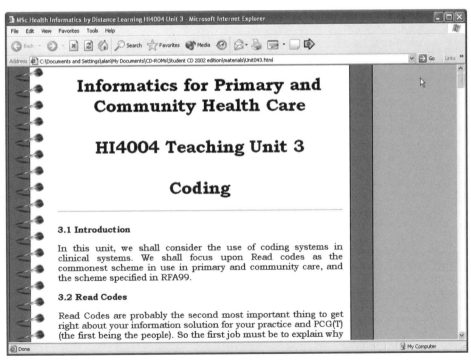

With the current developments in e-learning within the NHS under the banner of the NHS-U (the official name of the proposed NHS 'university'), this technology offers the NHS the chance to provide tailored learning programmes for every staff member.

This is either a utopian or Orwellian vision of the future. The utopian view goes something like this:

- it provides a convenient method of education for NHS staff
- it provides education which is relevant and necessary
- it provides high-quality education accredited by the NHS
- it provides economies of scale, allowing cost-effective provision.

The Orwellian view goes something like this:

- it provides a vehicle for training NHS staff in their own time
- it restricts training to that approved by the Government
- it provides training controlled by the NHS
- it is a high-visibility IT project which is never cost-effective in the NHS environment.

It is left to the reader to decide upon their own level of paranoia!

References

American Psychiatric Association (1980) *Diagnostic and Statistical Manual on Mental Disorders* (3e). American Psychiatric Association, Washington DC.

An Bord Altranais (2000a) *Requirements and Standards for Nurse Registration Education Programmes*. An Bord Altranais, Dublin.

An Bord Altranais (2000b) *Scope of Nursing and Midwifery Practice Framework*. An Bord Altranais, Dublin.

Beaumont G (1996) *Review of 100 NVQs/SVQs*. NCVQ/SCOTVEC, London.

Bedford H, Phillips T, Robinson J and Schostak J (1993) *Assessing Competencies in Nursing and Midwifery Education. The ACE Project*. ENB, London.

Benner P (1984) *From Novice to Expert: excellence and power in clinical nursing practice*. Addison Wesley, California.

Bentley TJ (1996) *Bridging the Performance Gap*. Gower, Aldershot.

Blackburn, Hyndburn and Ribble Valley NHS Trust (2000) *Building Trust and Confidence Among Staff and Patients for Equality, Equity, Diversity and Fair Treatment*. BHRV NHS Trust, Blackburn.

Blackburn, Hyndburn and Ribble Valley NHS Trust (2001) *Nursing and Midwifery Strategy – 2001–2004*. BHRV NHS Trust, Blackburn.

Care Sector Consortium (1989) *Draft Occupational Standards in Care*. CSC, London.

Cleckley H (1976) *The Mask of Sanity* (6e). Mosby, St Louis.

Confederation of British Industry (1994) *Quality Assessed: the CBI review of NVQs and SVQs*. CBI, London.

Conroy M (1996) *The Future Healthcare Workforce*. HSMU, Manchester.

Crosby PB (1979) *Quality is Free*. McGraw-Hill, London.

Department of Health (1994) *Nursing, Midwifery and Health-visiting Education: a statement of strategic intent*. DoH, London.

Department of Health (1997) *The New NHS*. HMSO, London.

Department of Health (1998a) *Information for Health*. HMSO, London.

Department of Health (1998b) *A First Class Service*. Department of Health, London.

Department of Health (1999) *Making a Difference*. Department of Health, Leeds.

Department of Health (2000a) *The NHS Plan*. Department of Health, Leeds.

Department of Health (2000b) *A Health Service of All the Talents: developing the NHS workforce*. Consultation document on the review of workforce planning. Department of Health, London.

Department of Health (2000c) *The NHS Plan: building the information core*. HMSO, London.

Dolan B and Coid J (1992) *Psychopathic and Antisocial Disorders: treatment and research issues*. Gaskell, London.

Dreyfus SE and Dreyfus HL (1980) *A Five-stage Model of the Mental Activities Involved in Skill Acquisition*. Unpublished report supported by the Air Force Office of Scientific Research. USAF, University of California, Berkeley.

Dymott S (1994) Speech to RCN Society of Occupational Health Nursing, Annual Conference. *Nursing Standard*. **8**(12): 7.

Eaton A (1994) Taken further to task over NVQs. Letter in Viewpoint section. *Nursing Standard*. **8**(12): 41.

Eraut M (1994) *Developing Professional Knowledge and Competence*. Falmer Press, London.

Eraut M (1998) Concepts of competence. *Journal of Interprofessional Care*. **12**(2): 127–39.

Eraut M (2001) *Keynote Paper at the Fifth International Conference on the Regulation of Nursing and Midwifery*. Copenhagen, Denmark, 8 June 2001.

Eraut M and Cole G (1993) *Assessing Competence in the Professions*. Research and Development Series, Report No. 14. Department of Employment, Sheffield.

Gilchrist JM (1992) Project evaluation using the SEI method. *Software Quality Journal*. **1**: 37–44.

Hare RD (1980) A research scale for the assessment of psychopathy in criminal populations. *Personality and Individual Differences*. **1**: 111–19.

Hare RD, Harpur TJ, Forth AE *et al.* (1990) The Revised Psychopathy Checklist: reliability and factor structure. Psychological assessment. *Journal of Consulting and Clinical Psychology*. **2**: 338–41.

Hogston R (1993) From competent novice to competent expert: a discussion of competence in the light of the post registration and practice project (PREPP). *Nurse Education Today*. **13**(3): 167–71.

Humphrey WS (1987) *Characterising the Software Process: a maturity framework*. Software Engineering Institute, CMU/SEI-87-TR-11, DTIC number ADA182895.

Humphrey WS (1989) *Managing the Software Process*. Addison-Wesley, Reading, MA.

Humphrey WS and Sweet WL (1987) *A Method for Assessing the Software Engineering Capability of Contractors*. Software Engineering Institute, CMU/SEI-87-TR-23, DTIC number ADA187320.

International Council of Nurses (1997) *ICN on Regulation: towards 21st century models*. ICN, Geneva.

International Council of Nurses (2001) *International Competencies for the Generalist Nurse*. ICN, Geneva.

Jessup J (1991) *Outcomes: NVQs and the emerging model of education and training*. Department of Employment, Sheffield.

Mansfield R and Mitchell L (1996) *Towards a Competent Workforce.* Gower, London.

McAllister M (1998) Competency standards: clarifying the issues. *Contemporary Nurse.* **7**: 131–7.

Melia P (1997) *Written Submission to the Judicial Inquiry.* Ashworth Hospital Authority, Merseyside.

Mitchell L (1998) *Models of Competence.* Paper presented at the RCN Vocational Qualification Forum Conference, 5 October 1998, Liverpool.

National Council for Vocational Qualifications (1989) *The NVQ Criteria and Related Guidance.* NCVQ, London.

National Council for Vocational Qualifications (1995) *NCVQ: the global pathfinder for vocational reform.* NCVQ, London.

NHS Executive (1999) *Agenda for Change.* NHS Executive, Leeds.

NHS Executive (2000) *Report of the External Review into Oxford Cardiac Services.* NHS Executive, SE Regional Office.

NHS Executive (2001) *Report of the Inquiry into Bristol Royal Infirmary.* NHS Executive, Leeds.

NHSIA (2001) *National Health Informatics Competency Profile.* The Stationery Office, London. Available online at www.nhsia.nhs.uk.

Nursing Board for Northern Ireland (2000) *Assessment of Practice.* Occasional Papers. NBNI, Belfast.

Nursing Board for Scotland (1995) *Competence to Practice: a literature review on competence to practice.* NBS, Edinburgh.

Oakes J (1994) There's no need to envy NVQs. Letter in Viewpoint section. *Nursing Standard.* **8**(16): 40–1.

O'Hanlon M and Andrews D (1997) Occupational standards: a framework for clinical effectiveness? *Nursing Management.* **3**(5): 24–6.

Parker S (1996) *Do Competence-based Approaches Have a Place in Higher Education? NVQ higher level competence and academic knowledge: are they compatible?* Conference proceedings, Universities Association for Continuing Education, Leeds, p. 39.

Paulk MC (1995) The evolution of SEI's Capability Maturity Model. *Software Process: improvement and practice.* **1**: 3–15.

Paulk MC, Curtis W, Chrissis MB and Weber CV (1991) *Capability Maturity Model for Software.* Software Engineering Institute, CMU/SEI-91-TR-24, DTIC number ADA240603.

Paulk MC, Curtis W, Chrissis MB and Weber CV (1993a) *Capability Maturity Model for Software, version 1.1.* Software Engineering Institute, CMU/SEI-93-TR-24, DTIC number ADA263403.

Paulk MC, Weber CV, Garcia SM, Chrissis MB and Bush MW (1993b) *Key Practices of the Capability Maturity Model, version 1.1.* Software Engineering Institute, CMU/SEI-93-TR-25, DTIC number ADA263432.

Professional and Practice Development Forum Scotland (1997) *Definition of Clinical Competence.* Unpublished.

Radice RA, Harding JT, Munnis PE and Philips RW (1985) A programming process study. *IBM Systems Journal.* **24**(2).

Royal College of Nursing (1994) *Educational Investment Portfolio.* Royal College of Nursing, London.

Shepherd G (1996) Announcement to the House of Commons when establishing the Committee of Enquiry into Higher Education in February 1996.

Stephenson J (1993) *Capability and Competences: are they the same and does it matter?* HEC, Leeds.

Storey L (1996) Portfolio development made easy. *Care Standard.* 10–13.

Storey L (1998) Functional analysis and occupational standards: their role in curriculum development. *Nurse Education Today.* **18**(1): 3–11.

Storey L (2001) *Providing Secure Nursing Care: a comparative study of services in the UK and Australia.* Florence Nightingale Foundation, London.

Storey L, Dale C and Martin M (1997) Social therapy: a developing model of care. *NT Research.* **2**(3): 210–18.

Storey L, Greenham S and Martin E (1995a) NVQs as part of the pre-registration diploma. *Nursing Times.* **91**(7): 34–5.

Storey L, O'Kell S and Day M (1995b) *Utilising National Occupational Standards as a Complement to Nursing Curricula.* NHS Executive, Leeds.

Storey L and Haigh C (2002) Portfolios in professional practice. *Nurse Education in Practice.* **March**.

UKCC (1992) *Code of Professional Practice.* UKCC, London.

UKCC (1999a) *Fitness for Practice. Report of the Commission into Nurse Education.* UKCC, London.

UKCC (1999b) *Standards for a Higher Level of Practice.* UKCC, London.

UKCC and University of Central Lancashire (1999) *Nursing in Secure Environments.* UKCC, London.

Universities Association for Continuing Education (1996) *The Purposes of Continuing Education.* Conference proceedings, UACE, Leeds.

Weber CV, Paulk MC, Wise CJ and Withey JV (1991) *Key Practices of the Capability Maturity Model.* Software Engineering Institute, CMU/SEI-91-TR-25, DTIC number ADA240604.

White EM (1994) Cited in: L Black, D Daiker, J Summers and G Stygall (eds) *New Directions in Portfolio Assessment.* Boynton/Cook Publishers, Heinemann, London.

Wolf A (1994) Assessing the broad skills within occupational competence. *Competence & Assessment.* **25**: 3–6.

World Health Organization (1988) *Learning to Work Together for Health. Report of a WHO study group on multi-professional education for health personnel: a team approach.* WHO, Switzerland.

World Health Organization (2001) *Nurses and Midwives for Health: WHO European strategy for nursing and midwifery education.* Guidelines Section 2: Competency-based education and training. WHO, Copenhagen.

Wright P (1993) *NVQs, GNVQs and NETTs: implications for universities and their staff.* Universities' Staff Development Unit, USDU Briefing, September 1993.

Further reading

Ashworth Hospital Authority (1997) *Written Submission to the Judicial Inquiry*. Ashworth Hospital Authority, Merseyside.

Beattie A (1987) Making a curriculum work. In: P Allen and M Jolly (eds) *The Curriculum in Nursing Education*. Croom Helm, London.

Day M and Basford L (1993) *Occupational Competence and Capability as a Complement to Professional Preparation: an assessment strategy for a Project 2000 Nurse Training Programme*. Sheffield & North Trent College of Nursing and Midwifery and University of Sheffield.

Dearing R (1996) *Review of Qualifications for 16–19 Year Olds*. SCAA, London.

Department for Education and Employment (1995) *HE Projects, Briefing Paper*. DfEE, Sheffield.

Department of Health (1989) *Caring for People*. DoH, London.

Department of Health (1991) *The Patients' Charter*. DoH, London.

Department of Health (1992) *The Health of the Nation*. DoH, London.

Department of Health (1993) *A Vision for the Future*. DoH, London.

Department of Health (1995) *Non-Medical Education and Training Planning Guidance for 1996/97*. EL(95)96. DoH, London.

Department of Health (1996) *Primary Care: the future*. HMSO, London.

Department of Health and Social Security (1977) *The National Health Service Act*. HMSO, London.

Dolan B (1996) *Perspectives on the Henderson Clinic*. The Henderson Clinic, Sutton.

Duffield C (1993) The Delphi technique: a comparison of results obtained using two expert panels. *International Journal of Nursing Studies*. **30**(3): 227–37.

Edwards C (1996) Within the framework. *The IHSM Network*. **3**(14): 6.

Employment Department (1993) *A Vision for Higher Level NVQs*. Employment Department, Sheffield.

Employment Department (1993) *Knowledge and Understanding: its place in relation to NVQs and SVQs*. Competence and Assessment Briefing Series. Employment Department, Sheffield.

Gillies AC (1998) Can computers improve the health of the nation? *Journal of Health Informatics*. **4**(2): 147–53.

Gillies AC (1998) Computers and the NHS: an analysis of their contribution to the past, present and future delivery of the National Health Service. *Journal of Information Technology*. **13**(8).

Gillies AC (2000) Assessing and improving the quality of information for health evaluation and promotion. *Methods of Information in Medicine*. **39**(3): 208–12.

Higher Education Quality Council (1995) *Vocational Qualifications and Standards in Focus*. HEQC, London.

Ministry of Justice (1991) *TBS (a special measure within the criminal code)*. Zorn Publishing Company, Leiden.

Paulk MC (1995) How ISO 9001 compares with the CMM. *IEEE Software*. **12**(1): 74–83.

Paulk MC and Garcia SM (1994) The impact of evolving the Capability Maturity Model to version 1.1. *Crosstalk: The Journal of Defence Software Engineering*. **7**(9): 7–11.

Paulk MC, Konrad MD and Garcia SM (1995) *CMM versus SPICE Architectures*. Software Process Newsletter, IEEE Technical Committee on Software Engineering.

Rhodes G and Charlton J (1996) *Where Do NVQs Fit into Universities?* Conference proceedings, Universities Association for Continuing Education, Leeds.

Storey L (1991) Viewpoint. *Nursing Standard*. **March 6**.

Storey L (2001) *The Concept of Competence*. Proceedings of Competence in Clinical Practice conference. An Bord Altranais, Dublin, September 2001.

Storey L and Dale C (1998) Meeting the needs of patients with personality disorders. *Mental Health Practice*. **1**(5): 20–6.

UKCC (1995) *Standards for Post-registration Education and Practice*. UKCC, London.

White E (1991) *The Future of Psychiatric Nursing by the Year 2000: a Delphi study*. University of Manchester.

Zopf S (1994) *Improvement of Software Development through ISO 9001 Certification and SEI Assessment. Software quality: concern for people*. Proceedings of the 4th European Software Quality Conference, pp. 224–231. VDF, Zurich.

Index